"This book is an important entry into th̲̲̲̲̲̲̲̲̲̲̲̲̲̲̲̲̲̲̲̲̲̲
care. The diverse perspectives and experience of the contributors will enrich the current understanding of what palliative care is and what it can be, even as it provokes a deeper and more textured discussion. Much of the focus of this volume, and what makes it a particularly valuable addition to a professional conversation that has been ongoing for more than thirty years, is the role that spirituality and religion play in palliative care, as they apply to better individual and social understanding of illness, of wellness and well-being, of mindfulness, and of relationships, particularly between providers, patients, and their families. Pegoraro and Benton are to be commended."

– MC Sullivan, RN, MTS, JD, chief healthcare ethicist,
Archdiocese of Boston

"This ambitious volume is akin to a woven tapestry that draws the reader into the critical and interconnected concepts that comprise spirituality, dignity, and palliative care. The collaborative and layered approach brings the readers through an exploration of intrapersonal, interpersonal, institutional, community, and public-policy factors that comprise a normative vision for palliative care, and the varied barriers that must be overcome to realize that goal. That vision is rendered vivid and practical through the use of powerful stories of patients and families facing illness, a diverse array of spiritual and religious perspectives, and evocative discussion questions. This book is a key resource for palliative care trainees, practitioners, and advocates."

– Tracy A. Balboni, MD, MPH, FAAHPM, associate professor of
radiation oncology, Harvard Medical School; clinical director,
The Supportive and Palliative Radiation Oncology Service,
Dana-Farber/Brigham and Women's Cancer Center

"In the world beyond cure, everyone is a pilgrim and every path is individual and personal. The deeply thoughtful and carefully researched chapters in this book offer all travelers both the enduring wisdom of the world's major faith traditions and the powerful psychological insights and interactive tools of today's medicine. *Finding Dignity at the End of Life* is a light in the darkness for those who travel to an unknown and deeply personal destination and those who accompany them to the edge of the world, whether we share their path because of professional competence or because of our love."

– Rachel Naomi Remen, MD, professor of medicine,
Boonshoft School of Medicine; clinical professor of family
and community medicine, UCSF School of Medicine

"A new tool for palliative care advocacy is here. Kathleen Benton and Renzo Pegoraro gather for us the voices of different cultures, religions, and practical approaches to palliative care. In the middle of different traditions and practices we can find the harmony of people caring in a holistic, compassionate, and respectful way for those that are in the critical moment of advanced disease and facing the end of their life. But the book is not only to recommend or promote palliative care. It is a practical roadmap, offering key points to those helping anyone in the spiritual process of saying goodbye. Relatives, caregivers, chaplains, and health professionals will enjoy reading through the pages of this book."

– **Professor Carlos Centeno Cortés**, head researcher, Atlantes Research Group, Institute of Culture and Society, University of Navarra

Finding Dignity at the End of Life

Finding Dignity at the End of Life discusses the need for palliative care as a human right and explores a whole-person methodology for use in treatment.

The book examines the concept of palliative care as a holistic human right from the perspective of multiple aspects of faith, ideology, culture, and nationality. Integrating a humanities-based approach, chapters provide detailed discussions of spirituality, suffering, and healing from scholars from around the world. Within each chapter, the authors address a different cultural and religious focus by examining how this topic relates to questions of inherent dignity, both ethically and theologically, and how different spiritual lenses may inform our interpretation of medical outcomes.

Mental health practitioners, allied professionals, and theologians will find this a useful and reflective guide to palliative care and its connection to faith, spirituality, and culture.

Kathleen Benton is president and CEO for Hospice Savannah, Inc. She is an experienced clinical ethicist and palliative care director with a history of working in the hospital and healthcare industry.

Renzo Pegoraro is a doctor, moral theologian, and bioethicist. He is chancellor of the Pontifical Academy for Life and professor of bioethics at the Faculty of Theology, Univeristy of Padua.

Finding Dignity at the End of Life

A Spiritual Reflection on Palliative Care

Edited by Kathleen Benton and Renzo Pegoraro

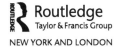

NEW YORK AND LONDON

First published 2021
by Routledge
52 Vanderbilt Avenue, New York, NY 10017

and by Routledge
2 Park Square, Milton Park, Abingdon, Oxon, OX14 4RN

Routledge is an imprint of the Taylor & Francis Group, an informa business

Library of Congress Cataloging-in-Publication Data
Names: Benton, Kathleen, editor. | Pegoraro, Renzo, editor.
Title: Finding dignity at the end of life : a spiritual reflection
   on palliative care / edited by Kathleen Benton and Renzo
   Pegoraro.
Description: New York, NY : Routledge, 2020. | Includes
   bibliographical references and index.
Identifiers: LCCN 2020014519 (print) | LCCN 2020014520
   (ebook) | ISBN 9780367206598 (hardback) | ISBN
   9780367206581 (paperback) | ISBN 9780429280252 (ebook)
Subjects: LCSH: Palliative treatment—Religious aspects. |
   Terminal care—Religious aspects. | Dignity.
Classification: LCC R726.8 .F5527 2020 (print) | LCC R726.8
   (ebook) | DDC 616.02/9—dc23
LC record available at https://lccn.loc.gov/2020014519
LC ebook record available at https://lccn.loc.gov/2020014520

ISBN: 978-0-367-20659-8 (hbk)
ISBN: 978-0-367-20658-1 (pbk)
ISBN: 978-0-429-28025-2 (ebk)

Typeset in Times New Roman
by Apex CoVantage, LLC

Contents

Tables and Figures

Tables

Figures

About the Contributors

Dr. Denisha Allicock, DrPH, MPH, serves as Project Director for a community organization under a non-profit organization. Her research interest is in Mental Health, Delivery Health Service, Advanced Care Planning, Palliative Care, Organization Performance and Assessment.

Dr. Ursula Bates is Principal Chartered Clinical Psychologist, Head of Psychology, Our Lady's Hospice and Care Services, Harold's Cross, Dublin.

Dr. Franca Benini MD is Director of Pediatric Palliative Care – Pain Service, Department of Women's and Children's Health, at the University of Padua in Italy.

Dr. Kathleen Benton is the President and CEO for a local Savannah-area hospice and palliative care organization. Prior to this appointment, she served as the Director of Ethics and Palliative Care at St. Joseph's/Candler Hospital for over a decade.

Dr. Eduardo Bruera, MD, is a hospice and palliative medicine specialist in Houston, Texas. He graduated from University Nac De Rosario Faculty De Med and specializes in hospice and palliative medicine.

Dr. Ferdinando Cancelli, MD, is Medical Doctor at Fondazione F.A.R.O. (home and hospice palliative care) in Onlus, Torino, Italy. Dr. Cancelli is a journalist for Osservatore Romano, Rome.

Dr. Carlo Casalone, MD, STD, is a Member of the Scientific Section of the Pontifical Academy for Life.

Eric Coles, MPA, is Doctor of Public Health Candidate at Harvard University.

Dr. Azza Adel Hassan is the Head of the Palliative Care Unit/Program Director, National Center for Cancer Care and Research, at Hamad Medical Corporation in Doha, Qatar.

Dr. Sister Nuala Patricia Kenny received an MD from Dalhousie University in 1972. She has received five Honorary Doctorates and in 1999 was appointed an Officer of the Order of Canada for her contributions to child health and medical education. Dr. Kenny is internationally recognized as an educator and physician ethicist.

Dr. Howard K. Koh is the Harvey V. Fineberg Professor of the Practice of Public Health Leadership at the Harvard T. H. Chan School of Public Health and the Harvard Kennedy School, as well as Faculty Co-Chair of the Harvard Advanced Leadership Initiative.

Hun Lee is a JD Candidate and was a Coordinator for the WHO Collaborating Centre for Training in Hospice & Palliative Care in Seoul, South Korea.

Dr. Emmanuel Luyirika, M FAM MED, MPA, BPA, MB, ChB, is Executive Director of the African Palliative Care Association (APCA), a membership organization with 4013 individual members and 1300 institutional members.

Dr. Mark E. Murphy, MD, FACP, AGAF, founded the Center for Digestive and Liver Health along with Dr. Rydzak in 1994. His principal clinical interests are in Crohn's disease, ulcerative colitis, liver disease, gastrointestinal malignancy, and advanced therapeutic endoscopy.

Dr. Srivieng Pairojkul, MD, is Associate Professor at the Department of Pediatrics, Faculty of Medicine, at Khon Kaen University and an Adjunct Associate Professor, Department of Pediatrics, Case Western Reserve University, USA.

Rev. Renzo Pegoraro, MD, is a doctor, moral theologian, and bioethicist. He is chancellor of the Pontifical Academy for Life and professor of bioethics at the Faculty of Theology, University of Padua.

Dr. Katherine Pettus is the Advocacy Officer for Palliative Care at International Association for Hospice & Palliative Care (IAHPC). She holds a PhD in Political Theory from Columbia University and a Masters in Health Law from the University of California San Diego. She also is a Freelance Translator and Editor, Latin American Scholarly Services.

Dr. Sara Plaspohl, DrPH, is Associate Dean for Waters College of Health Professions at Georgia Southern University.

Dr. Christina M. Puchalski, MD, MS, FACP, FAAHPM, is a pioneer and international leader in the movement to integrate spirituality into healthcare in clinical settings and medical education. She founded and is the Director of the George Washington Institute for Spirituality and Health (GWish). She is also Professor of Medicine at the George Washington University in Washington, DC.

Dr. Seema Rajesh Rao, MBBS, DPM, is Senior Medical Officer, Respite Palliative Care Project, at Dr Ernest Borges Memorial Home, Bandra. She is the Clinical and Administrative Head of the 13-bed inpatient respite care facility for palliative care patients from Tata Memorial Hospital.

Dr. Azar Naveen Saleem is Clinical Fellow in Palliative Medicine, National Center for Cancer Care & Research, at Hamad Medical Corporation in Doha, Qatar.

David Shannon is Senior Chartered Counselling Psychologist, Our Lady's Hospice and Care Services, Harold's Cross, Dublin.

Dr. Rabbi Nadia Siritsky, MSSW, BCC, is the Vice President of Mission of a large interfaith hospital system, Kentucky One Health in Louisville, Kentucky. She has worked as an interfaith chaplain and a psychotherapist in several settings, including hospice and palliative care.

Dr. Kimberson Tanco, MD, is Assistant Professor, University of Texas, MD Anderson Cancer Center, in Houston, Texas. He received his medical degree in 2005 from the University of Santo Tomas in Manila, Philippines, and did his Internal Medicine training at St. John's Episcopal Hospital, Far Rockaway, New York.

Denise C. Thompson, BCC, MBA, MAPS, is Chaplain at Memorial Health University Medical Center, Savannah, Georgia.

Dr. Vidya Viswanath, MD, is Assistant Professor in Palliative Care at Homi Bhabha Cancer Hospital and Research Center in Aganampudi, Visakhapatnam. She also volunteers as a Palliative Care Physician at St Josephs Hospice – the only hospice in the state of Andhra, Pradesh.

Dr. Jinsun (Sr. Julianna) Yong, PhD, RN, is Professor and Director, the WHO Collaborating Centre for Training in Hospice & Palliative Care, College of Nursing, the Catholic University of Korea, Seoul, South Korea.

Preface

A Voice of Community: Bringing Together the Ideologies to Form Congruence in Medicine

Palliative care can be a ground of consensus among different religious traditions and worldviews. In fact, it addresses fundamental health needs and issues concerning the ultimate questions about how people want to live and to die. Since these aspects of human life are universally felt as crucial, they can become a motivation for social cohesion. However, this cannot happen without a wide public debate in order to develop awareness, create the availability to collaborate, and ensure the ability to sustain the correspondent financial choices at a policy level.

Collaboration is a transversal aspect. First, it involves teams working in an interdisciplinary setting, given the complexity of the needs that are to be addressed – which highly technological biomedicine frequently neglects, since it is not well equipped to assume a holistic care of the person. Second, collaboration is needed between specific healthcare delivery systems and families, which are an asset of the network; following the situations of persons, particularly the elderly and the dying, in need of long-term care at home is both humanizing and economically more affordable. Finally, collaboration is promoted among the numerous stakeholders involved in the process at institutional and international levels.

The palliative care ethos challenges our contemporary global health ideology, which is fixated on making populations fit into a predetermined path and discarding those who cannot walk that path.

Patients treated in healthcare every day define one care, one life, one outcome. Evidence-based clinical medicine works hard to envelop these patients in groups defined by common diseases, common side effects, and common outcomes. This is necessary for science to achieve $n = $ a number worthy of making sense of a recommendation for many and to defend the use of a specific intervention or to justify the more challenging goal of defining some prognostic expectation. As scientifically driven humans, we hope to know what will happen; we try to discover and predict. However, the spiritual, religious, and peace-seeking minds of individual patients are too different to align with the aforementioned modern medical process. Thus, in this book, our experts concentrate on the trinity of areas we aim to advise on: religion, spirituality, and dignity.

These three areas are all interwoven components of good palliative care. This is the symptom control, the artful conversation, and the gatekeeping necessary to walk a patient and caregiver through illness. Palliative care is not mutually exclusive to aggressive care but rather supports and is a partner to concurrent treatment options.

This book presents a collection of disparate philosophies, traditions, beliefs or nonbeliefs, and ultimately a representation of the myriad of mentalities that weigh heavily into spirituality in medicine during suffering, chronic illness, and the terminal disease process when patients cling to something . . . unknown . . . and bigger. . .

As clinicians and healthcare givers walking with patients, their communities, their organizational backgrounds, and their interpersonal beliefs must be at least basically understood to reflect and offer soul-seeking peace. The authors' hope is that this book will serve as a reference for patients and their caregivers when curative healing is no longer an option.

Renzo Pegoraro, MD,
with Kathleen Benton, DrPH, MA

Part 1

Religion, Spirituality, and Palliative Care

Chapter 1

Defining Death Through Individual-Level Determinants

Denisha Allicock, Kathleen Benton, and Sara Plaspohl

This chapter serves as an introduction to the reader, highlighting the common thread among all individuals – despite their rooted or inherited belief system – that throughout disease, there is a universal need to find purpose and peace as a component of comfort, alluding to treatment. Further, the reader will see how the greater the organizational and community influences on a patient, the more likely they are to struggle with a personal or surrogate dilemma of choice in clinical care decisions.

As mentioned by the authors in the preface, patient beliefs must be understood to reflect and offer soul-seeking peace. A social ecological model is utilized to contextualize the theoretical framework of various reflections on palliative care. This model is based on work by theorists including Urie Bronfenbrenner (1977, 1979) and McLeroy, Bibeau, Steckler, and Glanz (1988), all of whom propose that behavior is shaped due to multiple levels of influence. There are five major levels of influence: intrapersonal, interpersonal, institutional, community, and public policy.

The innermost level of this layered approach includes *intrapersonal/individual factors* such as knowledge, attitudes, behavior, self-concept, skill, and developmental history, incorporating characteristics such as the individual's age, gender, sexual orientation, racial/ethnic identity, religious identity, and health literacy.

Moving outward, the next level of the ecological approach includes *interpersonal/social groups*. These groups may be formal networks such as co-workers, advisors, and supervisors or informal collections of family, friends, club/organization members, neighbors, and church members. These groups provide basic support systems for the individual.

The third level in this model includes *institutional/organizational factors* such as formal and informal rules and regulations. Examples may include policies and procedures for various clinical providers such as hospitals, nursing homes, physician offices, and hospice organizations.

The next level pertains to *community factors* characterized by relationships among organizations and institutions within defined boundaries. Formal groups such as businesses, community leaders, civic organizations, public health organizations, and care providers interact in various ways to serve the overall needs of the local community.

The outermost level of a social ecological model includes *public policy*. Local, state, and national jurisdictions maintain an array of laws and policies that define and guide the overall environment and behavior of the people at the various levels of governance.

The first section of this book focuses on the innermost core of the social ecological model (intrapersonal/individual factors), offering case studies and descriptions of people based upon geography and religion, highlighting similarities and differences among these populations with regard to how each views palliative care. Each patient is a unique and complex blend of knowledge, attitudes, behavior, self-concept, skills, and developmental history, influenced significantly by an array of personal traits. Many of these traits are demographic variables that are predetermined at birth, including age, gender, and racial/ethnic identity (see Table 1.1). Other factors such as sexual orientation, religious identity, and health literacy are more controllable by personal preferences and

Table 1.1 Socio-Ecological Factors.

Chapter	Palliative Care Perspective	Application of Social Ecological Characteristics
Chapter 2: Finding Dignity at the End-of-Life Through Palliative Care, Everywhere: A Spiritual Reflection on a Clinical Area	Location-Based: Thailand perspective	Age, gender, ethnic identity, religious identity, knowledge, behavior, family, attitudes, health literacy, developmental history
Chapter 3: Cultural Factors Enriching Palliative Care in the Middle East	Location-Based: Middle Eastern perspective	Age, gender, ethnic identity, religious identity, health literacy, family
Chapter 4: A Jewish Understanding of Palliative Care: Reclaiming the Health Process	Religion-Based: Jewish perspective	Religious identity, health literacy, family
Chapter 5: Palliative Care: A Hindu Perspective	Religion-Based: Hindu perspective	Religious identity, health literacy, family
Chapter 6: Palliative Care: A Christian Perspective	Religion-Based: Christian perspective	Religious identity, health literacy, family
Chapter 7: A Nontraditional Spirituality Perspective on Palliative Care	Religion-Based: Nontraditional spirituality perspective	Religious identity, health literacy, family

choice. Although the focus will be on intrapersonal/individual factors, the reader will quickly realize how the other levels in the model influence and interact with the innermost core factors of patients as they consider and receive palliative care. It will be evident how the patient's social network of family and friends, physical environment, and cultural values/norms within their community influence their beliefs and choices.

Religion is a set of beliefs, feelings, dogmas, and practices that define the relations between a human being and sacred divinity. It may be defined by practices, traditions, virtue/faith, or a unity in a community who share the same faith, such as a church. There is large variation in the rites, doctrines, and practices across the world. In fact, 89 percent of worldwide populations report an alignment with religion, and 75 percent consider this group very important to life decisions (VanderWeele, Balboni, & Koh, 2017).

Spirituality can be an ambiguous term but reflects what ultimate meaning and values there are in one's life, who one is, and what life is about. It does not imply a definitive higher power or omnipotent being but rather a deep sense of defining life.

Dignity is a subjective term, defined differently for each individual and rooted in a sense of feeling of worth. For some, it is independence. For others, it is the ability to communicate. Still for others, it is something indefinable but inherent in the soul's view of the self. Pain can remove dignity for some, while the lack of ability to communicate can remove it from others.

The soulful purpose of life, in whatever form, plays an important role in many people's lives. Subsequently, as individuals are near the end of life, they draw from their religious or spiritual connection to make decisions. A study of patients with lung cancer noted that faith was the second most important factor influencing treatment decisions (Phelps et al., 2009).

Palliative care is discussed here as the common solution and a necessary variable to achieve dignity, despite whatever religious or spiritual affiliation the patient has, if any. An artful and holistic discussion of pain, boundaries to aggressive care, and necessary elements for individual quality of life, the specialty of palliation aims to bring humanity back to the forefront of artful healing.

Unfortunately, policy, payers, and insurance are interwoven into the right for this care. Emergent care does not include a dying right for palliation or comfort. It remains an unexplained anomaly that patients who are terminally ill can access artificial support and continued, unlimited resuscitation that will likely be futile. However, a patient who needs symptom control, regular assessment of factors affecting quality of life, and an artful conversation may have a difficult time having it paid for under a government or private payer system.

It is the right of the human to have all these needs met, the right to have soul-seeking peace when illness and disease overtake the physiological being? – these are public health inherent rights, and thus the struggle itself is as multilayered and as complex as the palliative patient.

It is not uncommon to find that in many healthcare consortiums, systems, and the literature itself, ethics is aligned with palliative care (Krouse, Easson, & Angelos, 2003). Each reflects on issues of choice/autonomy and best interest at the end of life; thus, they are commonly interwoven. In a new study looking at ethical consults, the variable for spiritual or religious affiliation was examined as the core definition for association with the ethics consult population. Between 2014 and 2018, a total of 630 patients were referred to the Clinical Ethics and Palliative Care Committee. The patient data contained several demographic questions and medical histories. These questions included items on gender, age in years, race, marital status, primary language, religious association, ZIP code, vent status, do not resuscitate status, pre-plan, and insurance. The majority of the patients were religious (69 percent, $n = 469$), while 31 percent ($n = 211$) were nonreligious. A faith background was the most common alignment among all analyzed ethics consults over the four years.

In this environment, an ethics consult is defined by a dilemma involved with clinical treatment decisions. It can be called by any member of the team, including family, though most were triggered by the involved physician. Reasons for a consult included many variables; thus, variation is evident throughout this set of four-year data. However, most of the cases involved critically ill, and potentially terminally ill, patients alluding to the ethical issues surrounding a decision about treatment in the final phase of illness or life. For the purpose of the data analysis, the description of the characteristics was aggregated by religious association. These data were computed as percentages of the total number of cases for each year with a combined summative frequency. In summary, the data showed that patients who were religious tended to struggle to die with dignity compared to patients who were not associated with religious preference. This led to asking the question: Is a strong belief system a catalyst to difficult decision-making at the end of life?

The simple variable of being part of an organization with some moral life teachings aligned the patients with the ethical dilemma of one choice or another. It did not matter the tradition or nontradition, however one may define it. The variable that mattered in four years of ethics consult data was simply the presence of religion in the patient's demographic. Very close to 100 percent of the patients examined over four years of data declared some tradition on their face sheet at the hospital.

Table 1.2 Religious Preference of Patients.

	Frequency	Percent
Religion preference	469	69.0
None/unknown religious	211	31.0
Total	680	100.0

An ethical dilemma, put simply, was warranted when the clinical staff disagreed with the family or the patient on what clinical steps should be taken next before the decision was made. If the physician is making a decision for long-term life support or resuscitation, the menu list of what end of life can look like is presented on a platter for the patient/family to decide. And suddenly conflict occurs. Literature supports the claim that those with religion have a more difficult time making logical, scientifically driven end-of-life decisions (Romain & Sprung, 2014). Whether there is the fear of judgment from a higher power or the steady patience for a "miracle" to occur may be two of many considerations. In anecdotal conversations with people, a focus-group question of what would be expected shows that people assume those with a religion would embrace the end of life in a more spiritual, hopeful, and life-eternal perspective. However, research says otherwise. Those with no tie to tradition or religion, in fact, account for fewer ethical dilemmas than the former, at least during the four years of data previously – thus proving that the actual moral tradition, belief system, or habits of praise and worship matter not. It is instead the tie to something higher than the self that leads to conflict at the end and a pull to artificial supports and away from allowing a natural death to occur. The data in this chapter show that ethical issues in medicine could be reflective of an alignment with a cultural or religious boundary. Exploring different perspectives surrounding the struggle with an acceptance for palliation and what is allowable within the confines of a person's moral compass lead to the same interpersonal struggles.

Medicine is disjointed. Differences are found in the way a specialist chooses to treat an illness and in the inability of those specialists to communicate with one another. Spiritual healing even among different value systems requires a more similar protocol for all. It may not be the same because two patients are simply members of the same area of faith. It may not be the same because one has, or lacks, belief. Within each belief system, there are divisions among divisions, and no one person can align with any single other person. Thus, the best we can do as healthcare givers is to understand some existential version of those beliefs and support our patients in their walk. The best that all caregivers can do is to embody holistic care.

The continuum of care shown in Figure 1.1 portrays a line with the extremes of care at each end, euthanasia-like comfort at one end and aggressive care at the other, noting that the biggest area is the gray; the gray explores that there is no final decision that can be made for or against a belief system in the face of disease. Interpretation, personal beliefs, burden, and level of suffering must all be considered in placing a patient on this continuum. Though state, federal, and universal policies aim to address the extreme ends, it is the middle section that will serve most patients as they walk through disease.

All interwoven components of good palliative care include symptom control and the artful conversation and gatekeeping necessary to walk a patient and caregiver through illness, not mutually exclusive to aggressive care but

Euthanasia
Assisted Suicide

Full Aggressive
Artificial Support

Figure 1.1 Continuum of Care at End of Life.

rather concurrent with and working as a gatekeeper in detailed explanation of every organ working with the diagnosed illness, in contrast to explanation of only the organ of the specialist's expertise. Palliative care firmly embraces the multilayered interworkings of the layered model (Pask et al., 2018). Further, the Institute of Medicine (2014) cites that one of the important assessments for a patient in palliative need is their spiritual well-being and outlook, a key determinant of complex levels of suffering. Despite the number of protocols present for a curative effort toward illness, there are no standard definitions for what may constitute the complexity of a progressively ill person. Access of palliative care is not determined by this complexity. Rather, access is usually a result of the given specialist's understanding for the need to palliate. An integrated care model, considering a person's macrosystem, their microsystem, their environment, and their support, is a constant in the presence of pain and suffering. The Holistic Common Assessment tool lends scientific truth to the anomaly of mental and spiritual pain present in disease (NHS National End of Life Care Programme, 2010). A patient must have some ability to cope, to mentally cling to hope, or to have some idea of finding purpose or explanation in illness. This could potentially be a burdensome concept for a patient with no tradition, no group, no belonging spiritually or even further complicated by the diverse intercollections among the continuity of one ideology. This collection seeks to discover meaning sought in different ways adding up to one universal truth.

As clinicians and healthcare givers walking with patients, the patient's community, their organizational background, and their interpersonal beliefs must be at least basically understood to reflect and offer soul-seeking peace. The authors' hope is that this book will serve as a reference for those patients, family members, and caregivers that one might turn to when curative healing is no longer an option

Palliative care as defined by the National Hospice and Palliative Care Organization (2019) can occur in any setting from home to nursing home, clinic, or hospital. Palliative patients pursue "curative treatment modalities" and do not relinquish aggressive or artificial measures. However, with palliative care as a component, the focus is upstream of a six-month prognosis and works in congruence to assess serious symptoms, relieve stress, and navigate options with support from a team beyond just clinicians into chaplaincy and social services. Palliative patients are complex from mentality to physicality; there is not one universal definition of who may benefit from palliative care, but what is universal is the integrated nature in which palliative specialists work to address multilayered issues. This book unfolds into a varied portrayal of beliefs and practices, for it is impossible for it all to gel into one single method given our human differences. For many years, technology and specialists have replaced physician–patient rapport and good discussion. With the art of new treatment, it is quite possible that the art of being human was lost within medicine. As human beings, we are much more than our physical self, much more than the shell of the person; we are a spirit and a soul. Many spirits are fed by something deeper than this world has to offer and thus that must be nurtured and tended. This is not defined necessarily by an organizational religion or a specific spirituality but rather the idea that as humans, we are complex. As treatments are "done to" us, our whole self may seem less tended to than is required to achieve dignity. In essence, we stopped relying on medicine to treat our soul. Yet the soul is the full actualization of the being (Shields, 2016), so without treating the being, we are inherently denying the right of the soul. Protocols, procedures, anatomy, and biology are inherent to the curriculum of the healer. But as caregivers, we must not forget to school our learning clinicians and support staff in healing when biologic life is at its end phase. After all, as caregivers, we only have one chance to get someone's end of life right.

Discussion Questions

1. How can this model/perspective be used in practice to understand patient end-of-life care needs in different settings?
2. How would you apply the socio-ecological model to accomplish a prevention or promotional change in behaviors during end of life for palliative care and health workers?
3. What are some additional determinants that influence end-of-life care at the individual level?
4. What are some additional determinants that influence end-of-life care at the interpersonal level?
5. What are some additional determinants that influence end-of-life care at the organization level?
6. What are some additional determinants that influence end-of-life care at the community level?
7. What are some additional determinants that influence end-of-life care at the policy level?

References

Bronfenbrenner, U. (1977). Toward an experimental ecology of human development. *American Psychologist* 32, 513–531.

Bronfenbrenner, U. (1979). *The Ecology of Human Development.* Cambridge, MA: Harvard University Press.

Krouse, R., Easson, A., & Angelos, P. (2003). Ethical considerations and barriers to research in surgical palliative care. *Ethics and Barriers to Research in Palliative Care* 196(3), 469–474.

McLeroy, K., Bibeau, D., Steckler, A., & Glanz, K. (1988). An ecological perspective on health promotion programs. *Health Education Quarterly* 15(4), 351–377.

National Hospice and Palliative Care Organization. (2019). Explanation of palliative care. www.nhpco.org/palliative-care-overview/explanation-of-palliative-care/.

NHS National End of Life Care Programme. (2010). Holistic common assessment of the supportive and palliative care needs of adults requiring end of life care. www.bl.uk/collection-items/holistic-common-assessment-of-the-supportive-and-palliative-care-needs-of-adults-requiring-end-of-life-care.

Pask, S., Pinto, C., Bristowe, K., Vliet, L., Nicholson, C., Evans, C., . . . Murtagh, F. (2018). A framework for complexity in palliative care: A qualitative study with patients, family carers, and professionals. *Palliative Medicine* 32(6), 1078–1090.

Phelps, A. C., Maciejewski, P. K., Nilsson, M., Balboni, T. A., Wright, A. A., Paulk, M. E., . . . Prigerson, H. G. (2009). Religious coping and use of intensive life-prolonging care near death in patients with advanced cancer. *Journal of the American Medical Association* 11, 1140–1147. doi:10.1001/jama.2009.341.

Romain, M., & Sprung, C. L. (2014). End-of-life practices in the intensive care unit: The importance of geography, religion, religious affiliation, and culture. *Rambam Maimonides Medical Journal* 5(1), e0003. doi:10.5041/RMMJ.10137.

Shields, C. (2016). Aristotle's psychology. In E. N. Zalta (Ed.), *The Stanford Encyclopedia of Philosophy.* https://plato.stanford.edu/archives/win2016/entries/aristotle-psychology/.

VanderWeele, T. J., Balboni, T., & Koh, H. (2017). Health and spirituality. *Journal of the American Medical Association* 318(6), 519–520. doi:10.1001/jama.2017.8136.

Chapter 2

Finding Dignity at the End of Life Through Palliative Care Everywhere

A Spiritual Reflection on a Clinical Area

Srivieng Pairojkul

> *As stated earlier, palliative care means treating the patient in the environ-ment in which he or she is most comfortable, maintaining the traditions and beliefs the patient prefers as much as possible in a medical setting. It also sometimes involves family members who share different beliefs and requires that we find a way to merge their preferences so that all who participate in the end-of-life care, including the patient, find a way to let go without vio-lating their most deeply held longings.*

As palliative physicians, even if we only have a short time to get to know our patients, we are able to get to know them truly well. We know who they are, what they are like, what their beliefs and values are. We walk along with our patients and their families, be with them, take care of them with respect. Each patient leaves an imprint in our memories. We are grateful that they have given us a chance to understand how valuable life is, as well as how sacred is death. All we do is help them live with the best possible quality of life and die with dignity.

Case Study No. 1: Choosing to Let Go

Ice, a 16-year-old, was admitted to the Pediatric Intensive Care Unit (PICU) in Thailand for nearly two months and was referred to us for withdrawal of her life support. The first time I met her was two weeks before the consulta-tion, when I went into the PICU to see another patient. I walked past her bed and saw a distressed girl, both hands restrained to the bed. I asked the nurse, "Why do you have to tie her?" The nurse answered, "She had pulled out her endotracheal tube twice, so we need to restrain her." Ice looked sad, and both of her eyelids were puffy. I learned that she had systemic lupus erythematosus (SLE) that was resistant to all treatment, and now she had septic shock with acute respiratory distress syndrome. I couldn't dig more into her history at the time, since the primary doctor had consulted us on another case. I felt pity for her, since from her condition, she should have been receiving our services. Two weeks later, we received another case consultation from the PICU, and this time, the patient was Ice. The reason for the consultation was that all the pediatric specialists suggested that nothing could be done for her. Her SLE treatment was resistant to corticosteroids and chemotherapy, and she had commenced peritoneal dialysis due to renal failure from nephropathy. She had been admitted to the PICU several times due to pneumonia off and on, and this time was the worst. She had hospital-acquired pneumonia and neutropenia, complicated with septic shock, and later developed acute respiratory distress syndrome (ARDS). The pediatric infectious specialist stated that her infection could not be controlled even with the most effective antibiotics and that she now also had a fungal infection. She was put on a mechanical ventilator due to respiratory failure. It seemed that Ice recognized that this was her end, and she wanted to end her own suffering. She had pulled out the endotracheal tube twice, but each time, she was reintubated and both her hands were restrained. When she developed pulmonary edema, her pediatric chest specialist wanted to try her on high-pressure treatment, hoping to keep her alive. After tremendous treatment, all the doctors agreed that nothing could be done and that they wanted to seek help from the palliative care team.

I visited her this next time with my nurse. I introduced myself to her and told her that we were there for her to provide her comfort and to be her companions. She was fully conscious but needed to communicate with yes-or-no questions and sometimes wrote what she wanted. She pointed to the endotracheal tube and gave signs that she wanted to take it out. She wrote, "Let me go." I realized that if I took the endotracheal tube out, she would die in minutes or perhaps hours. She was receiving high oxygen and high pressure and was on a high dose of inotropes. I told her that if I took the tube out, she would die in a short time. She nodded her head to give me a signal that she knew that. I told her that I needed to talk with her parents and that they needed to sign the consent form. I asked her if there was anything else she wanted me to do for her. These were her wishes: She wanted to donate her body to the medical faculty and to have last rites (merit) from a Buddhist monk. She told us that she had nothing to give back to society except her body. Her other wishes were to have a chance to taste her favorite food, which was an omelet; she wanted to be dressed in a pink dress, which was her favorite color; and she wanted to see her father, whom she had not seen since she was a small child. I promised her that I would try my best to respond to all her wishes.

My nurse managed to make an appointment with Ice's mother. She had lived in another province since her divorce 10 years earlier and had remarried a man who was a construction worker, with whom she had two more children. She had left her first two daughters (Ice and her sister) with her parents, who were farmers. Ice's father had not seen his daughters for a very long time and had never sent any support; he had also remarried and lived in another province.

Ice's mother visited her daughters from time to time and sent money to support the children.

We had a chance to listen to Ice's story and came to know her well. She was very responsible, growing up on her own. She was mature and had taken good care of herself and her sister. At age 13, she had been diagnosed with SLE, which required regular visits to the hospital. She came to the hospital by herself and followed the appointment schedule regularly. Unfortunately, it seemed her SLE was poorly responsive to corticosteroids and chemotherapy, and her kidney function deteriorated to the point that she needed peritoneal dialysis. She also had to be admitted several times due to infections. Her carers were her younger sister and grandmother. Her sister helped with managing the dialysis at night. Both Ice and her sister still attended school. At one point, Ice had to quit school due to frequent admissions to the hospital. Ice had taught her sister to be honest and generous. When the disease became poorly controlled, she told her sister to behave well if she was not there to take care of her anymore. She mentioned that everybody must die – it's the nature of life – that she was prepared for her imminent death, and she was not afraid.

We informed Ice's mother that her condition was serious and that she was dying. We mentioned to her that Ice wanted to withdraw life support and prepare to die. Her mother, a tough, middle-aged woman, was crying and said that she felt guilty for not being able to raise her but agreed to her decision. She realized how much suffering Ice had endured during the past two months but that now it was time for her to rest peacefully. We consoled her and sat with her for a while; after signing the informed consent, she left to be with Ice in the PICU. Later that afternoon, I visited Ice and her mother and described to them the process of withdrawal of life support. I reassured her that we would effectively control her symptoms and that she would not suffer.

My nurse bought Ice a pink dress, and she also bought an omelet for her. We invited the monk to perform a praying ceremony at her bedside; then Ice gave the offering dedicated to the monk. The whole time, she was calm and looked peaceful. I gave her a small piece of omelet to let her taste her favorite food after having tasted nothing for two months. Later I asked her, "Are you ready, Ice?" She nodded her head, received a kiss from her mother and sister, and then we extubated her. I whispered in her ear, "Ice, you are now free of all the pain and suffering. May all your good deeds provide you a better next life." We had responded to all her wishes, except the one wish that we could not achieve: seeing her father, who never came. Under sedation, she died peacefully with dignity after all life support was withdrawn. Her mother and her sister were by her side.

Since this was the first case in which we had withdrawn life support in the PICU, we then arranged a reflection session with the PICU nurses and the pediatric residents. According to Thai culture and religious beliefs, killing is a sin in Buddhism, and some people saw withholding/withdrawing life support as killing. The residents reflected that they felt uneasy, but if they had been the patient, they would have chosen what Ice did. The nurses were concerned that some might consider it a sin. I explained to them that Ice was dying and all the life support caused her suffering. She had autonomy to choose what she valued. We did not kill her, but we realized that even with all the life support, she would not survive, so we let go and let her die from the natural cause of the illness.

Case Study No. 2: Reunion

Duen, a beautiful 29-year-old woman, was referred to us by her surgeon. She had advanced breast cancer that had metastasized to her lungs and pleura. She struggled to live but could not resist the cancer.

Duen had been diagnosed with breast cancer three years earlier. She had a mastectomy and finished her chemotherapy with regular follow-ups. She worked as a receptionist for a car company and was beloved by her boss and her friends because she was sweet and cheerful. Her boyfriend supported her all the way through her cancer treatment. They decided to get married, hoping to start a happy family. One month after the marriage, Duen was admitted with breathing difficulty. The CT scan showed that she had lung metastasis, with fluid in her lung. A tube was inserted into her chest to drain the fluid. While she was treated in the hospital, she realized that she had missed her period, and the test showed that she was pregnant. Her primary doctor, a surgeon, suggested an abortion, since she might need chemotherapy to treat the recurrent cancer. It was a shock for the family. Only a month before, their lives had been full of happiness, and now the world was upside down for them. Duen decided to have the abortion, but she cried all day and night; she felt guilty for terminating her baby's life. The family had made a merit by going to the slaughterhouse and saving a cow from being killed. Thai culture allows one to save one's life by making a good merit. One week after the abortion, Duen had a high fever, and an antibiotic was started to treat her pneumonia. Two weeks later, the fever still persisted despite changing the antibiotic. The fluid in her lung was now loculated, and the chest tube was taken out. Duen was now in despair; she had been admitted for a month, had lost her baby, and her condition was run down. Chemotherapy could not be started due to her infection and her lessening function. The palliative care team was consulted, and on the day that we saw her, she told the doctor that she wanted to go back home for several days because she was too stressed and needed a break. A psychiatrist had been consulted to see her after the abortion, and she had been put on an antidepressant. We had only talked with her on the day that she was discharged home. We told her that we wanted to help her with her breathlessness symptom and that we would be with her all the way through her illness. Morphine was started to control her symptoms. She came back again two days later with difficulty breathing and required oxygen therapy. We realized that she would die soon. The chest x-ray showed progression of lung metastasis, with loculated effusion.

Duen's mother was a nurse and worked in a nearby province. We informed her that Duen's condition was serious and that her time was short. We asked if Duen knew her prognosis. We hadn't explored her understanding of her condition because on the day that we saw Duen before she was discharged, she was very distressed and we thought we could do the advance care planning when she came back. Duen's family was in a state of shock, and they agreed with me that we should inform Duen so that she could be prepared and that we needed to talk about comfort care.

In Thai culture, the doctor does not inform the patient directly about the prognosis, and the palliative consultation usually comes late. The primary care team can feel uneasy informing a patient or family of bad news and often leaves it to the palliative care team to disclose the truth to them. We controlled Duen's symptoms with subcutaneous morphine and midazolam. We then disclosed her prognosis to her and said that at some point, if she was too breathless, we would need to increase the medication. Duen listened to us in a quiet manner. She cried, but it seemed she was coping very well. Later on, Duen stayed quietly with her mother and husband. She asked her mother to sing her a lullaby so that when she joined her baby, she would sing a lullaby for her. All her family – her mother, husband, and sister – stayed by her side. She died peacefully two days later.

Case Study No. 3: Acceptance of Destiny

A 24-year-old man struggled to live without knowing his prognosis. His wife and family knew the prognosis, but they were still looking for a miracle and encouraged him to endure the suffering so that he could have a chance to live. When the palliative care team got involved, after informing the family that he would not survive, we asked that the patient be told about the prognosis. Finally, the family acceded. We talked with the patient and informed him about his situation, whereupon the patient cried in agony. Finally, he accepted his destiny. We reassured him that we would relieve him of all the pain and all suffering. Even if his condition could not be cured, he would be looked after to provide comfort care. He died peacefully the next morning. It seems that he realized that it was time to let go, and he lost energy abruptly.

Case Study No. 4: Searching for Miracles

Boonsong, a 41-year-old man, was admitted to the isolation room in the cardiac ICU for one month. The cardiologist consulted us because he could do nothing for the patient. Boonsong had been diagnosed with end-stage kidney disease at the age of 16. He received a kidney transplant and had been well until nine years earlier when he had graft rejection; he then switched to hemodialysis two times per week. One month prior to this admission, he developed dyspnea and leg swelling, was admitted to a private hospital, and then was referred to our hospital because he had cardiac tamponade from massive peri-cardial effusion and volume overload. He was admitted to the cardiac ICU, and a pericardial window was performed. Unfortunately, he developed bacterial pericarditis and later on was intubated and put on a ventilator. His course was complicated with septic shock and gastrointestinal bleeding, which required multiple blood transfusions. He did not respond to antibiotics but developed a multidrug-resistant strain and fungal infection. He needed platelet transfusion due to bleeding and platelet consumption. Hemodialysis was still continued while he received inotropes to maintain his blood pressure. At this point, the cardiologist, infectious disease specialist, and nephrologist suggested that the treatment should be stopped. The palliative care team was sent in to manage the situation and also care for the patient and his family.

Boonsong had one son from his first marriage, which ended in divorce. He married a second time and lived with his second wife. They were supported by his well-to-do family financially, since Boonsong needed medical treat-ment, and he was very well taken care of by his wife and family. During his admission, his wife visited him every day, but since he had been infected with resistant bacteria, he needed to stay in an isolation room and only short visits were allowed. His wife cheered him up and made him promise that he would not lose hope and that he would fight very hard for her. At this stage, the fam-ily still insisted to the care team that they wanted everything to be done and refused to stop treatment. The family was looking for a miracle.

When I first visited him, I saw a cachexic man looking distressed. His skin was full of bleeding spots and patches and needle stick marks. I realized that his time was short and that he would never leave the ICU. I gathered that while he was sick in the ICU, he had never had a chance to see himself. His general condition was so poor, there were several lines and five or six infusion pumps around him. He did not have the energy to raise his hand to write. I told him that we were a palliative care team. Our duty was to help him by managing all the symptoms that distressed him. I informed him that his condition was seri-ous, but he frowned and shook his head. I understood that he was not happy to hear what I had said. He then turned his face away from me and made a signal that he did not want to talk with me. I told him that we would visit him and be with him. We asked the ward nurse about Boonsong's family. The information that we got was that his wife visited him regularly. Every time, she would cry and ask Boonsong to fight for her. She could not live without him. Boonsong was the eldest son, with three younger sisters, who also visited him regularly. After our first visit, I told my nurse to explore the family and get to know more about the patient. We made an appointment to meet with the family on the next day.

A family meeting was conducted with Boonsong's wife, his three sis-ters, and his mother. I informed the family of the objectives of the meeting, then explored the family structure and relationship. This was a warm fam-ily, and everybody was concerned about Boonsong. I explored the family's understanding of Boonsong's condition. They all knew that it was serious, but they hoped for a miracle and they wanted the care team to do everything. They stated that Boonsong was a fighter: He had fought with his kidney disease since he was a teenager, had gone through all the treatments, and had never lost hope. I disclosed to the family the grave prognosis that he would never leave the ICU. The family were all crying and tried to support Boonsong's wife. I tried to guide the family to see all the suffering that he had to endure and that it was time to relieve him from all suffering and let him go. All the current treatments were not working anymore, and they would only create suffering. I made another appointment to meet with the family again in the next two days. I told the ward nurse to let the wife spend more time with Boonsong and help with the nursing care. Before this, every time his wife had visited him, it was after the nurse had finished his bed bath and snugged him under the blanket, which hid all the marks of his suffering.

The second meeting was quite smooth. The family stated that they wanted to stop his suffering. The family expressed that never before had they looked closely at Boonsong's condition. After they helped with the nursing care and saw his body and observed him choking when being suctioned from the endotracheal tube, they saw how much suffering Boonsong had to endure, and they wanted to end it. The family asked me to talk to Boonsong and to disclose the prognosis to him. I came to talk with Boonsong. I told him that I had talked with his wife and his family about his situation. They all realized how much suffering he had gone through. They knew that all the time, he had fought for them. I told him that I thought he would not be able to leave the ICU, and I suggested that we should choose comfort care. The family came in and told him that he could let go; they loved him so much that they did not want him to suffer any more. All the time while he listened to me and later to his family, he cried in agony; later, though, in a calm state, he nodded his head to show that he understood. The family stayed with him in the ICU. Dialysis and ino-tropes and antibiotics were withdrawn, and he died peacefully on that day sur-rounded by his family. I called the family a week later after they had finished the funeral. They were still feeling sad, but felt relief that they had released Boonsong from all the suffering. They said thank you for what we had done, and they wished the cardiologist had consulted our team earlier.

Case Study No. 5: Memories

Wanpen, a 24-year-old pregnant woman, had an ultrasound done at 20 weeks gestation. The obstetrician told the family that the fetus might have a severe heart defect and that it might not survive. The family's grief started from that day. A multidisciplinary team meeting was triggered with a fetal medicine spe-cialist, a neonatologist, a pediatric cardiologist, a cardiac surgeon, and the pal-liative care team. The diagnosis was single ventricle. After a family meeting, the family decided to continue the pregnancy, with support from the palliative care team. The parents had good support from their families. The father felt guilty, and he related the incident to sins committed in the past when, many years earlier, he had enjoyed going to the forest to shoot birds. We told him that the incident was nobody's fault: It was an accident. We continued to support the parents, a birth plan was discussed, and the parents decided not to do resuscitation in case the baby was distressed. The family had been informed of the baby's condition and that the surgical correction for the cardiac defect was risky. The family decided to choose comfort care for the baby. On the delivery day, the mother gave birth to a beautiful baby, and he looked healthy. They knew that they would have several days with the baby. We put the family in a special room, helping the parents to keep memoirs of their baby. They did the baby's hand and foot printing and the baby's photo and nurtured the baby. They had a chance to parent the baby only for a few days before the baby became respiratorily distressed, was diagnosed with cyanosis, and later died peacefully under morphine infusion to help relieve the symptoms. Their grief still continued, but the parents knew that they had given their baby love and comfort and that this memory would remain with them forever.

Case Study No. 6: Bonding

One time I had a chance to teach pediatric palliative care to a group of nurses. I mentioned the perinatal palliative program that we had organized and told them this case. In the northeast of Thailand, where I work, I came across a mother who had delivered a baby who was not compatible with life. The grandmother would not allow the mother to see the baby for fear that it would create psychological trauma and break the bond between mother and child. While I was talking about this issue, one nurse went out from the lecture room. I thought she might have gone to the restroom. Later this nurse came back and walked to the microphone. She said she wanted to express something. She told us that she had given birth to an abnormal baby, and when she listened to the story of my patient, it triggered her emotions, and she went out of the lecture room to cry. She shared with us her experience. After recovering from a Caesarean section, her husband came to tell her that their baby had severe anomalies and was dying. He told her that she should not see the baby, thinking that she could not cope. The baby died a day later. That nurse cried and expressed her feelings. She felt guilty that she had not given her baby love and comfort. If she could turn back time, she wanted to hold her baby in her arms and give it comfort and unconditional love, even if only for a little while. All the participants gave her support. We have provided support for several families through our perinatal palliative care program and come across several cases where grandparents did not want the parents to form an attachment to their dying newborn baby. They thought that it would prevent the parents from unsettled grief, but from our experience, it was the instinct of the parents to have unconditional love for their dying babies. We try every means to let the parents see and hold their newborn babies, and we found that nothing could prevent them from bonding with their babies. The babies should not die alone. They should be held by their parents, who provide them with love and care until the baby's time comes.

Discussion Questions

1. Within the Thai community, how are key figures (family, physicians, and healthcare staff) impacted by palliative care?
2. What are some of the determining factors that may impact end-of-life care in the Thai community?

Chapter 3

Cultural Factors Enriching Palliative Care in the Middle East

Azar Naveen Saleem and Azza Adel Hassan

For many patients, religion is a part of their core being, and setting aside deeply held beliefs is near impossible. For Muslims, healthcare settings provide both a haven where care can be provided as well as a setting where compromises may need to be made when it comes to religious complications. Caught between the science of healthcare and the religious preferences of the patient, medical staff will find that knowing the patient's culture and religious rituals help them find the middle ground so that the patient's health is not sacrificed and religious beliefs are not violated.

The Region

The Middle East is a transcontinental region stretching across Western Asia. The history of the Middle East dates back to ancient times, with the geopolitical importance of the region being recognized for centuries (Shoup, 2011). The Middle East has played an important role in shaping the history of civilizations and nations. It's one of the vital centers of the globe religiously, socially, politically, and economically. There are 17 countries that make up the Middle East (World Population Review, 2019): Bahrain, Cyprus, Egypt, Iran, Iraq, Israel, Jordan, Kuwait, Lebanon, Oman, Palestine, Qatar, Saudi Arabia, Syria, Turkey, United Arab Emirates, and Yemen. Out of the 17 countries, Saudi Arabia is the largest country in the region and Bahrain the smallest. Arabs, Turks, Persians, Kurds, and Azeris (excluding Azerbaijan) constitute the largest ethnic groups in the region by population, with Arabs constituting the largest ethnic group in the region by a clear margin.

The Middle East is multicultural and multireligious. Most of the major religions that are practiced around the world have their origins in the Middle East. This includes Judaism, Christianity, and Islam. It is also believed that most of the messengers who came with the revelation from God belong to the same geographical location.

Presently, Islam is the largest religion in the Middle East, representing approximately 95 percent of the total population in the region (Exhibition, 2017). About 20 percent of the world's Muslims live in the Middle East (Pew

Research Center, 2009). Islam is a monotheistic faith, with the cornerstone being faith in Allah, the one single god. A Muslim is a person who follows the religion of Islam. Muslims follow the teachings of the holy text, the Quran, which is believed to be the revelation from God himself that was revealed through the messenger of God, the Prophet Mohammed (Peace be upon him).[1] The followers of Islam believe that the Prophet Mohammed (PBUH) was the last of the messengers sent by God to Earth. A Muslim also believes in the prophecies given to all the prophets, including Adam, Moses, and Jesus.

The Middle East has a population of over 411 million people (World Population Review, 2019). The population in the Middle East has been growing steadily with advancements in healthcare, unlike some other regions where there has been a steady decline in population. Egypt is the most populated and Bahrain is the least populated country in the region.

Cancer is the second leading cause of death globally and was responsible for an estimated 9.6 million deaths in 2018. Globally, about one in six deaths is due to cancer. Approximately 70 percent of deaths from cancer occur in low- and middle-income countries (Cancer, 2018). The incidence of cancer has been steadily growing in the Middle Eastern region. The World Health Organization (WHO) estimated that in the Eastern Mediterranean region – which includes the Middle East – there were 555,318 new cases of cancer in 2012, and by 2030, this could rise to 961,098, meaning the Eastern Mediterranean will have the highest relative increase of all regions in the world (Rizvi, 2016). This is alarming, as the people dying of cancer also are also proportionately increasing in the region. In another 20 to 30 years, the region shall witness a substantial increase in the geriatric population, which demands a robust palliative and home healthcare system.

The Influence of Culture and Religion in the Region

The local culture is heavily based on and influenced by Islamic principles. The influence can be seen in day-to-day practices, interpersonal interactions, and decision-making in healthcare.

The discovery of petroleum and gas in the region revolutionized infrastructure and led to rapid economic growth over the past 50 years. Advancements in healthcare, research, standards of living, and economic development are currently on par with those of Western countries, although this varies from country to country within the region. However, the cultural and social ethos remains strongly rooted in tradition. In general, the size of families is much larger than what is observed in Western society.

The Holy Quran says, "and we sent down of the Quran that which is healing and mercy for the believers" (17:82), which means that those people who make the Quran their guide and book of law are favored with the blessings of Allah and are cured of all their mental, psychological, moral, and cultural diseases.

The Prophet Muhammad (PBUH) said, "No fatigue, no disease, no sorrow, no sadness, no hurt nor distress befalls a Muslim, even if it were a prick of a thorn, but Allah expiates some of his sins for that" (Sahih al Bukhari, Book 75, Hadith 2). This helps patients and families cope with illness and suffering.

There are various cultural norms and practices that play into the social dynamics of the region. These include rules governing gender interactions, preconceived notions regarding medications like opioids, a lack of patient autonomy, and shared decision-making affected by a patriarchal hierarchy. Though being culturally accepting of death, there is great reticence in withdrawing futile treatment even in the face of inevitable death. The most common social and cultural factors affecting healthcare in the region are enumerated subsequently.

Gender Interactions

Muslims have a prescribed set of rules and regulations regarding gender interactions. Males and females are required to practice a high level of modesty per the Islamic teachings, as evidenced by the verse in the Holy Quran, "Tell the believing men to lower their gaze and to be mindful of their chastity: this will be most conducive to their purity – [and,] verily, God is aware of all that they do. And tell the believing women to lower their gaze and to be mindful of their chastity, and not to display their charms [in public] beyond what may [decently] be apparent thereof" (Quran 24:30–31).

Men usually dress in a garment that covers the whole body and head except the hands and feet. The design and color vary among the different Middle Eastern countries. Women prefer to wear a cloak called *abayah* and a headscarf. A considerable percentage of women also prefer to cover their face.

Unlike in Western society, free interaction between the opposite sexes is discouraged. Usually, healthy gender segregation is the norm once children reach the age of adolescence. In Islam, any relationship with the opposite gender should be purposeful. The institution of marriage is highly respected, forms the basis of society, and is the only acceptable relationship between an unrelated man and woman. Even 1400 years ago, as the scriptures suggest, Muslim women held their dignity and were usually shy around men; however, they were confident enough to work and address men when necessary. The Quran and the teachings of Prophet Mohammed (PBUH) have highly emphasized respecting and protecting women. The etiquette and rules of gender interaction extend to all fields, which also includes healthcare.

Notions Regarding Modern Medications and Treatment Practices

The illicit use of recreational drugs, alcohol, and all forms of leisurely intoxicants are strictly prohibited in Islam. The Quran and the teachings of Prophet Mohammed (PBUH) have regarded intoxication as a sin. "O you who have believed, indeed, intoxicants, gambling, [sacrificing on] stone altars [to other than Allah], and divining arrows are but defilement from the work of Satan, so avoid it that you may be successful" (Quran 5:90).

Islam encourages Muslims to seek treatment for their illnesses. Easing the suffering of an individual is considered an admirable deed, but the majority of patients and families have preconceived misconceptions regarding medications like sedatives and narcotics, which necessitates a detailed explanation. The use of medications that can induce drowsiness and sleep is usually scrutinized by the patient and the family. Prescribed medications like opioids for pain control are considered permissible because of their need. Patients and families accept the use of opioids for symptom control if the indication for their use is clearly explained to them. It is important to explain to the patient and family the possible side effects, as there may be concerns regarding drowsiness or sedation. Muslim patients prefer to be alert for the sake of the mandatory prayers, which occur five times a day. In terminally ill or dying patients, it is difficult to maintain a state of balance allowing for optimal symptom control and a normal level of consciousness.

Patient Autonomy

Patient autonomy is one of the core principles guiding medical ethics. Personal autonomy is, at a minimum, self-rule that is free from both controlling interferences by others and from limitations, such as inadequate understanding, that prevent meaningful choice (Varelius, 2006). Unlike in the West, there is always more emphasis on family and society over the individual in the Middle East. This presents a unique set of challenges in shared decision-making. Usually, medical outcomes are discussed with family members of the patient rather than the patient themselves. The families of the patient may refuse to disclose the medical diagnosis to the patient, especially if the patient belongs to a pediatric or geriatric age group. This presents a great hindrance in involving the patients in the process of treatment. The rationale behind this is that the family thinks unfavorable outcomes may cause huge distress to the patient (for example, with a diagnosis of cancer). With the improvement in healthcare awareness, education, and research, the views of the young population in the region are changing. The willingness to make the patient participate in their medical decisions is generally improving within the newer generations, where we may find instances where the patient prefers to hide his or her condition from close relatives to avoid distress to them.

On the other hand, this may be seen as a reflection of the care and concern families have for patients. Illnesses are viewed as a collective burden rather than an individual's personal battle. Many people prefer to share the difficulties involved in undertaking complex healthcare decisions with their families, and some may avoid it altogether, reflecting their trust in their families. Patients tend to be quite well supported through their treatment process.

Cleanliness

Cleanliness is a very important aspect of Islam. The Quran and the teachings of the Prophet Mohammed (PBUH) emphasize the importance of cleanliness. Muslims have to undertake obligatory ritual washing before each prayer, and cleanliness is strongly encouraged at all times as an act of faith. In Islam, prayer is considered the most important pillar and considered mandatory in all circumstances. The Quran says,

> O you who have believed when you rise to [perform] prayer, wash your faces and your forearms to the elbows and wipe over your heads and wash your feet to the ankles. And if you are in a state of janabah,[2] then purify yourselves. But if you are ill or on a journey or one of you comes from the place of relieving himself or you have contacted women and do not find water, then seek clean earth and wipe over your faces and hands with it. Allah does not intend to make difficulty for you, but He intends to purify you and complete His favor upon you that you may be grateful.
>
> (Quran 5:6)

Oral hygiene through cleaning the teeth with the use of a form of toothbrush called *miswak* is considered a good deed. Ritual ablution is also very important, as observed by the practices of partial ablution (*wudhu*), full ablution (*gushl*), and water-free alternatives using any natural surface such as rock, sand, or dust (*tayammum*). In Middle Eastern countries, bathrooms are often equipped with a shower situated next to the toilet so that individuals may wash properly. This ablution is required in order to maintain ritual cleanliness. The common Muslim practice of taking off shoes when entering mosques and homes is also based on ritual cleanliness (Islamic hygienical jurisprudence, n.d.).

Fasting and the Holy Month of Ramadan

Muslims consider Ramadan a holy month. The teachings of Islam instruct all healthy adult males and females to fast during the whole month of Ramadan. Fasting is observed for a period of 30 days during which Muslims abstain from all forms of food and drink predawn to sunset. The Quran says, "O you who believe, fasting is prescribed for you as it was prescribed for those before you that you may become righteous" (Quran 2:183).

Muslims who fast are advised to be self disciplined and to abstain from any sinful act. Sick people, travelers, and pregnant women are exempted from fasting. According to the teachings of the faith, it is important for the believer to compensate for the fast at a later date if missed for the previous reasons, except in case of terminal illness. Still, the vast majority of Muslim patients prefer to fast during the month of Ramadan, which poses a unique challenge for health-care professionals in the region.

Visitors

Islam and Middle Eastern culture encourage visiting sick people. Various teachings of the Prophet Mohammed (PBUH) have emphasized the importance and benefits of visiting sick people. In the region, visiting the ill and afflicted is considered a good and virtuous deed. The Middle Eastern people believe that visiting the sick is one of the clear signs of mutual love and empathy. More than that, visiting the sick is a major responsibility that every single Muslim is duty bound to fulfill. This also has an implication in healthcare, especially palliative care, as the patients receive many visitors from their extended family. The hospital visitation policies are bound to be relaxed in the region for the very same reason.

Death, Burial, and Bereavement

Unlike Western culture, Middle Eastern people are more accepting of the notion of death as a society. Patients who are terminally ill and those in their dying phase prefer to be involved in prayers asking forgiveness from God; they also reach out to their family, friends, and acquaintances to ask forgiveness for all the intentional and unintentional mistakes that they may have made in life. In the palliative care setting, patients who are approaching death may even express their wish to perform the religious pilgrimage to the holy mosque of Mecca. The families of the patients try their best to make the patient's wish a reality. Unfulfilled wishes may cause great emotional distress to the family. Healthcare professionals should be cognizant of this fact and need to be supportive of the family in order to prevent potential feelings of guilt. Muslims believe in the concept of life after death. Usually, the family member who is caring for the patient during the time of death constantly reminds them to seek God's blessings and paradise. The caregivers also recite verses from the Quran during the death phase.

Family members expect the body of the deceased to be handled with care and dignity. An autopsy is generally refused by the family unless absolutely necessary for legal reasons or other investigations. The palliative care and healthcare teams are expected to express empathy to the family and to expedite the process of documentation and necessary paperwork after death. Per Islamic practice, burial and funeral formalities should be completed as soon as possible, ideally not exceeding 24 hours. The funeral prayer is usually performed by a large group of the Muslim community, many of whom will participate in the burial as well. Grieving by expression of compassion and shedding tears is common in the region. However, wailing and lamenting are prohibited. Bereavement follow-up may not always be necessary due to the strong family and community support in Middle Eastern society. However, the palliative care team may need to identify families with suboptimal resources and provide the necessary support during the bereavement period (Al-Shahri & Al-Khenaizan, 2005).

Palliative Care in the Region

Palliative care is an emerging branch of medicine in the Middle East. It was first introduced in Saudi Arabia in 1992, and countries such as Qatar, Kuwait, Jordan, Lebanon, Egypt, and the UAE already have progressive palliative care services. Cancer and other chronic diseases remain a major challenge for populations in the Middle East. About 50 to 60 percent of all patients with cancer in the region visit a physician for the first time when the tumor has reached advanced stages and is not curable. Palliative care and other active modalities play a vital role for those patients. There is a need for well-established fully functioning palliative care units to take care of such patients and alleviate their complaints. The effect of culture and the fact that families are more likely to place their patients in a hospital imposes the need for long-term services that are currently rare in the area. Home care and hospices are required in areas where hospital spaces are limited.

The Middle East Cancer Consortium (MECC), established in 1996, is a unique and valuable nongovernmental organization that works in Middle Eastern countries and collaborates with regional ministers of health and international healthcare organizations. Political issues, scarcity of resources, and lack of education and awareness seem to be the common factors restricting the progress of this field in most of the Middle Eastern countries. In order to improve the suboptimal palliative care services in the Middle East, emphasis should be directed toward providing formal education to professionals and raising awareness in the public. It is also necessary to put all differences aside and develop cross-border collaborations, whether through the World Health Organization, third-party organizations such as the Middle East Cancer Consortium, or others (Silberman, Daher, Fahmi-Abdalla, Jaloudi, & Hassan, 2015; Zeinah, Al-Kindi, & Hassan, 2012).

The inclusion of palliative care in the region's national healthcare strategy is a great step forward for the specialty in the Middle East. Many hospitals and institutions in the region have started fellowship programs, physician training programs, and nurse training programs in palliative care medicine. Palliative care and hospice development in the region will significantly improve the quality of life of dying patients with terminal illnesses. Most of the Middle Eastern countries, including the Gulf Cooperation Council (GCC) countries, are striving hard to establish palliative care services that deliver high-quality palliative care for patients with cancer. The aim is to achieve the best possible care for patients through the relief of suffering, control of pain and other distressing symptoms, and restoration of functional capacity while remaining sensitive to personal, cultural, and religious values and beliefs.

Clinical Challenges Due to Cultural and Religious Practices

There are significant challenges to effective clinical practice in the Middle East, as practice norms have to take into account the complexity of cultural and religious factors. As mentioned previously, healthcare practices and decisions are heavily influenced by local cultural and religious beliefs. The palliative care specialty faces further unique and difficult challenges in the region.

Treatment of palliative care patients often involves using sedatives and narcotics like opioids. This is often viewed with mistrust and often necessitates a detailed explanation on the part of the healthcare provider. There is often fear regarding opioid addiction.

One of the major challenges involved is the do not resuscitate (DNR) decision and discussion. Per Islamic teachings, all mentally competent adults of both genders are granted the full right to accept or refuse medical intervention. In reality, however, close family members often contribute significantly to the decision-making process. Generally, in Muslim families, the parents, spouses, and elder children, in descending order, have greater decision-making power than the rest of the relatives. This applies to DNR discussions also. The palliative care team is expected to have extended family meetings with or without the presence of the patient for treatment decisions (Al-Shahri & Al-Khenaizan, 2005). There are instances where the patient may not be involved in DNR decisions due to family insistence. Due to the lack of developed palliative care, hospice care, and home health services in the region, families of the dying patient prefer to keep the patient in the hospital setting for better medical and nursing care. The concept of euthanasia, which is the intentional ending of life to relieve pain and suffering, is not practiced and is considered prohibited in the region.

Muslim families are usually cynical about definitive responses from healthcare professionals. They are likely to be more comfortable with less definitive answers and may respond like, "This is in God's hands, and no one can predict anything." This is because Muslims believe that only God can determine the life span and time of death of every human being. Consequently, it is very difficult to get patients to put in place advance directives and plans.

The most important religious factors with healthcare implications include prayers and fasting. Adults are required to perform the obligatory five prayers a day. In spite of the space between each prayer and the permission for patients to combine some prayers to end up with three periods instead of five, many patients would prefer to continue performing prayers following the ritual public announcement (*Adhan*) for prayers heard from nearby mosques or on the television. Such patients would appreciate it if medical and nursing interventions could be avoided during these times. The patients need to face the Holy Mosque in Mecca during prayers, should that be possible. Assistance by members of the nursing staff would be appreciated for the patient who is not totally independent. Prayers involve certain movements, including standing, bowing from the waist, sitting, and kneeling. Patients who are unable to perform some or all of these movements are exempted. A quadriplegic patient, for instance, could perfectly perform prayers lying in bed. During prayers, the patients will neither answer questions nor attend to requests. Indeed, they would prefer the surrounding environment to be as quiet as possible.

Patients are usually exempted from fasting during the holy month of Ramadan, but there are considerable numbers of patients who continue fasting against medical advice and often do not appreciate healthcare professionals' recommendations. It is therefore advisable to leave the religious decisions to the family and the patient after explanation (Al-Shahri, 2002).

A vast majority of healthcare providers and staff belong to multicultural, multireligious, and multinational backgrounds. When people from such diverse groups are involved in patient care in the region, they are presented with numerous challenges. One of the major challenges is that healthcare professionals need to know the cultural and religious knowledge of the region.

Conclusion

Islamic principles heavily influence the culture and day-to-day practices of people in the Middle East. This is also reflected in the unique healthcare norms in the region and poses some specific and rather difficult challenges to the field of palliative care. A nuanced understanding of the various cultural and religious factors will enable healthcare professionals to understand patient perspectives and avoid conflict in order to enable effective delivery of quality care. Palliative care continues to grow rapidly in the region, and there is a need to fulfill the unmet needs in care delivery. Various programs aimed at training healthcare professionals are expected to improve the current void.

Discussion Questions

1. To what extent do Middle Eastern cultural norms impact quality of end-of-life care?
2. Can cultural norms impact the healthcare system?

Notes

1. In Islamic practice, the prophets are always addressed with respect, and it is customary to mention "peace be upon them/him" after their names.
2. The word *janabah* means "A state of major ritual impurity caused by any sexual contact." The state of *janabah* renders Muslims unfit for the performance of ritual duties, such as prayer, until they purify themselves through complete ablution (*ghusl*). "Janabah," s.v. Oxford Islamic Studies Online, www.oxfordislamicstudies.com/article/opr/t125/e1187.

References

Abu Zeinah, G. F., Al-Kindi, S. G., & Hassan, A. A. (2012, April). Middle East experience in palliative care. *American Journal of Hospice & Palliative Medicine* 30(1), 94–99. doi:10.1177/1049909112439619.

Al-Shahri, M. Z. (2002). Culturally sensitive caring for Saudi patients. *Journal of Transcultural Nursing* 13(2), 133–138.

Al-Shahri, M. Z., & Al-Khenaizan, A. (2005). Palliative care for Muslim patients. *Supportive Oncology* 3(6), 435.

Cancer. (2018). World Health Organization. www.who.int/news-room/fact-sheets/detail/cancer.

Exhibition. (2017). *Islam in Asia: Diversity in Past and Present: Muslim Populations*. Cornell University. http://guides.library.cornell.edu/IslamAsiaExhibit/Muslim Populations.

Islamic hygienical jurisprudence. (n.d.). Wikipedia. https://en.wikipedia.org/wiki/Islamic_hygienical_jurisprudence.

Pew Research Center. (2009). Mapping the global Muslim population. www.pewforum.org/2009/10/07/mapping-the-global-muslim-population/.

Rizvi, Anan. (2016). Middle East cancer rates expected to double in 20 years, says WHO. *National*. www.thenational.ae/uae/middle-east-cancer-rates-expected-to-double-in-20-years-says-who-1.199246.

Shoup, J. A. (2011). *Ethnic Groups of Africa and the Middle East: An Encyclopedia*. New York: ABC-CLIO.

Silbermann, M., Daher, M., Fahmi-Abdalla, R., Jaloudi, M. A., & Hassan, A. A. (2015, April). The Middle East Cancer Consortium promotes palliative care. *Lancet* 385(9978), 1620–1621. doi:10.1016/S0140-6736(15)60791-7.

Varelius, Jukka. (2006, December). The value of autonomy in medical ethics. *Medicine, Health Care, and Philosophy* 9(3), 377–388.

World Population Review. (2019, May). The Middle East population. http://worldpopulationreview.com/continents/the-middle-east/.

Chapter 4

A Jewish Understanding of Palliative Care

Reclaiming the Healing Process

Rabbi Nadia Siritsky

Among the myriad traditions in Jewish thought, the sanctity of life is ever present. There is a fine line between end-of-life care so that a patient is allowed to die with dignity without actively encouraging death and the prolonging of life at whatever cost necessary. With thousands of years of tradition, Judaism can draw upon its roots to allow patients, their families, and medical providers to balance scientific thought and religious training in a way that provides peace of mind to all.

In this chapter, we review the many texts and laws within Judaism that provide guidance and insight into the importance of end-of-life care as a means of honoring these Jewish principles. By exploring how this biblical teaching impacts Jewish teachings related to the relationships between medicine, prayer, and faith, the author focuses on their application in palliative and end-of-life care. We also explore the influence of the Holocaust upon Jewish theology related to meaning-making, suffering, and end-of-life issues.

One of the Hebrew words that is most commonly used around the world is: "L'chayim!" which is literally translated as "To life!" Frequently used as an expression of celebration, the affirmation of the inherent sanctity of life is a central tenet in Judaism – this despite the wide diversity of views, beliefs, and practices within Judaism.

The purpose of this chapter is to explore, within the body of traditional Jewish text, those sources and teachings that reflect the tonal understanding within Judaism regarding its affirmation of the sanctity of life and its understanding of palliative care.

These and These: Multiple Understandings of Truth

There is an old joke about Judaism: "two Jews, three opinions," although some would probably go so far as to say, "two Jews, ten opinions." This makes it challenging to write "what Jews believe about. . . " anything. There are multiple denominations and traditions within Judaism and multiple types of texts, some of which are *aggadic*, which is to say stories and parables that reflect certain enduring truths and principles, while others are *halachic*, which is to say legal compendiums and responsa designed to try to translate these truths into something concrete and tangible.

Many of these texts, both aggadic and halachic, contradict each other. This lack of consistency between rabbinic sources and interpretations of biblical texts is challenging when seeking guidance on a given topic but also reflects a deeper humility and recognition that the Truth that springs from the Eternal One is greater than all the truths that we have tried to glean in our attempt to make meaning out of our world and our experience.

The Hebrew bible has no vowels or punctuation in its original form. This leaves room for interpretation but also an awareness that all of our interpretations are both correct and incorrect, in that the multiplicity of interpretations contained in the original Hebrew may very well have been intended, in order to encourage the wrestling with meaning that is the essence of Jewish thought. This idea is contained in the name given to Jacob, and given to all of Jacob's progeny – namely, Yisrael, which is often translated as "one who wrestles with G!d."

Jews traditionally do not write out the Divine Name, recognizing that The Infinite Source of Creation and Blessing is beyond anything that our finite human minds and language can conceive. Many Jews write "G!d" as a way of expressing this belief, and for the purposes of this chapter, I have done this, too. With this practice comes a humility that all of our human understandings of G!d's Will are necessarily limited and imperfect.

This multiplicity of interpretations is most famously illustrated in the classic rabbinic story found in the Talmud, Eruvin 13b, which describes a series of arguments between two authoritative schools of rabbinic thought, Beit Hillel (the students of Hillel) and Beit Shammai (the students of Shammai). Ultimately, a Divine Voice ruled "these and these are both words of the Living G!d."

Indeed, the Talmud contains generations upon generations of rabbis, adding to the teachings of those who came before them, sometimes through aggadic text, story, and interpretation, and sometimes through halachic interpretation and legal thinking. These diverse perspectives continue to this very day; however, for the purpose of this chapter, both aggadic sources and halachic sources will be treated as sources of truth that provide glimpses into the enduring principles and values that can inform our question, namely: What is the tonal understanding within Judaism regarding the sanctity of life and the importance of palliative care?

Furthermore, although contemporary Jewish thinking has only expanded its historic diversity of interpretations of G!d's Will, with multiple denominations, each forming to seek to understand how ancient tradition is to be understood in our own day, this chapter references primarily Orthodox rabbinic scholars in their attempt to apply and preserve ancient teachings to contemporary issues in medicine.

Enduring Impact of Holocaust on Jewish Thought

It would be impossible to reflect upon Jewish beliefs concerning life, death, and Divine Will without acknowledging the impact that the Holocaust has had on contemporary Jewish theologians. The quest for meaning in the midst of suffering and the impulse for *pikuach nefesh* (the saving of a life), which undergirds so much of Jewish thought through the centuries, was tested most powerfully in the writings that emerged in the aftermath of this cataclysmic tragedy that exceeds human capacity to understand.

The Holocaust survivor and Austrian neurologist and psychiatrist Dr. Viktor E. Frankl stated:

> If there is a meaning in life at all, then there must be a meaning in suffering. Suffering is an eradicable part of life, even as fate and death. Without suffering and death, human life cannot be complete. The way in which a man accepts his fate, and all the suffering it entails, the way in which he takes up his cross, gives him ample opportunity – even under the most difficult of circumstances – to add a deeper meaning to his life. It may remain brave, dignified and unselfish. Or in the bitter fight for self-preservation, he may forget his human dignity and become no more than an animal.
>
> (Frankl, 2006)

This distinction between the dignity of the human being and self-preservation at all costs points to a dilemma that palliative care seeks to answer. The desire to avoid suffering, which often serves as an argument for assisted suicide, is not, according to this view, "compassionate." The suffering that is part of the dying process is not something to be avoided; rather, it is an integral part of life and an opportunity to "add a deeper meaning" to life.

Nevertheless, this requires a capacity to derive meaning in order to imbue one's existence with dignity and actualize the sanctity that is implanted within each person. Chaplaincy and spiritual care, which are important parts of the interdisciplinary team that provides palliative care, are uniquely skilled in assisting individuals to make meaning out of their experiences and, in so doing, to help them to achieve this developmental life task (Eilberg, 2001).

Caring for Life

Jewish tradition is replete with rituals and principles that reflect caring for life: from the tradition of giving monetary gifts in denominations of 18 (representing the numerical value of the Hebrew letters that spell out "chai" or "life") to the understanding that the most important Jewish laws, such as those related to the Sabbath, should be broken in order to save a life. Fundamental to this approach is the theological understanding that the truest expression of our faith is our grateful stewardship for the gift of life that we have been given.

The Hebrew bible's account of creation describes the Holy One breathing the Breath of Life into the nostrils of the first human. The implication is that the Soul-Breath that animates us contains Divine Breath: this Life Force therefore connects us with the Source of all Creation, and decisions that we make about our lives and our breath have profound theological implications. Indeed, Jewish mysticism affirms that all of creation contains Sparks of the Divine.

Emerging from these principles, Jewish tradition has a highly nuanced understanding of what G!d wants, which is drawn from centuries of rabbinic interpretation of the Written Torah (the first five books of Moses that comprise the Pentateuch) along with the Oral Torah, which was believed to have been passed down from generation to generation until it was finally written down in the Talmud. Others have come to understand rabbinic thought to be more reflective of a partnership between G!d and humans in attempting to speak Truth into human language. Either way, these texts provide the fertile ground from which Jewish thought derives.

This process of transcribing and preserving an ancient understanding of revelation and Divine Will is necessarily imperfect, limited by the inherent imperfection of human language and perception, and therefore subject to ongoing rabbinic debate as to how to adapt and interpret these principles in a modern-day world. As such, the one principle that guides discussions regarding the role of medicine in end-of-life decisions is the need to be cautious and to ensure that an overarching reverence for G!d and for life guides all such conversations.

This reverent caution can be seen in Jewish legal principles such as "the fence around the Torah," which seeks to create a type of legal guardrail around important Jewish laws in order to ensure that there not be any unintentional violation due to misinterpretation. It therefore follows that Judaism has traditionally rejected any legislation that advocates for active euthanasia or medically assisted death in its abundance of caution and reverence for the legal principle of *pikuach nefesh*, which refers to the importance of "saving a life" even if contraindicated by other important laws like Shabbat (the Sabbath).

Medicine: Partnering with G!d

Medical treatment is considered a sacred obligation, whereby we show our gratitude for the gift of life that we have been given. The legal compendium of the Shulchan Aruch, in Yoreh Deah 336:1, states that if a doctor refuses to heal, that doctor is guilty of bloodshed.

Indeed, while there is generally some division among Jewish legal scholars on most things, all agree that Jewish law mandates that a patient seek out medical care and that one has a duty to accept medical care in any situation where one has a reasonable expectation of recovery or at the very least of prolonging one's life and quality of life with treatment. This is based upon Deuteronomy 4:9, which commands one to *shmor nafshecha*, which can be translated as guarding one's life. The rabbinic commentary of Shevet Yehuda 336 states that those who do not go to doctors and accept the medical help that they need are acting with "criminal negligence" regarding their health and will have to stand on trial for this at the end of time.

It is also an obligation for the doctor to do everything possible to heal the patient, with the great medieval rabbi and physician Maimonides commenting on Deuteronomy 22:4, "you shall return it to him," that this teaches that doctors must do everything in their power to "return" to the patient all that he has lost, which includes the patient's health (Maimonides, 1168).

Care for those who are ill is a sacred obligation, and, indeed, all encounters with those who are sick are holy. The Talmud (Shabbat 12b) teaches that G!d's Presence hovers over the head of one who is ill. This has profound implications for the way we interact with those who are sick. When we enter into a patient's room, we are standing on holy ground.

If one were to reflect upon the implications of this teaching, we would recognize that medical care is a form of worship. We are entering into the Presence of G!d as soon as we enter the patient's room. The patient, created in the Divine Image, is breathing the Breath of Life, and it is the responsibility of the care team to ensure that this Sacred Energy and Life Force is able to be sustained in this world. Reverence ought to guide every medical decision and treatment.

Too often, traditional medical care loses sight of the fundamental holiness that is inherent in any conversation with a patient. Modern medicine depersonalizes the patient. We refer to the patient by their room number or diagnosis. We scan the patient like an item being purchased at a supermarket. We frequently consider cost and insurance as a deciding factor in the patient's care, as do patients themselves. We metaphorically dismember the patient, with one doctor focused on one organ, another on a different organ or specialty. Rarely within the traditional medical model do doctors or service line providers ever sit together with the patient to consider what this all means, nor do they consider the goals of care or priorities of the patient. Equally infrequent is a pastoral presence; although many hospitals do have chaplains, they are often called to provide spiritual care in a way that is not integrated with the rest of the care team. Overall, contemporary medicine tends to disempower and objectify the patient.

Judaism defines as idolatrous the objectification of that which is sourced in Divinity. The spiritual danger of modern medicine is that it will lose sight of the underlying mystery and sanctity through its focus on individual body parts and theories. By failing to engage in whole-person care, by failing to join with the patient or provide support, by failing to acknowledge the Presence of the Divine that is with the patient, modern medicine runs the risk of idolatry. It is precisely this reality that compels a reconsideration of the value of palliative care from the Jewish perspective.

Jewish Understandings of Palliative Care

Many people believe that palliative care is contrary to Jewish values, in part because of a misunderstanding of Jewish values and in part because of a misunderstanding of what palliative care is. Palliative care is frequently conflated with hospice, which is also frequently misunderstood.

The Center to Advance Palliative Care provides the following definition: "Palliative care is specialized medical care for people with serious illnesses. It is focused on providing patients with relief from the symptoms, pain, and stress of a serious illness – whatever the diagnosis. The goal is to improve quality of life for both the patient and the family" (National Palliative Care Research Center, n.d.).

Palliating symptoms of distress should be a fundamental goal of medicine. Doing so in a holistic and interdisciplinary manner ensures effective care that is both patient led and evidence based in its effectiveness. The research surrounding this statement is clear.

Research studies point to the improved patient experience and reduced pain and treatment complications of both palliative care and hospice. By focusing on the entire person and helping them access additional sources of support from their family and community, as well as from an interdisciplinary treatment team, patients generally live longer and require less expensive medical treatment than those with a similar diagnosis who undergo treatment from the traditional medical model.

Yet palliative care remains controversial. One may theorize that it is because it threatens the status quo of the healthcare system, which too often values profit over patient outcomes, or one may theorize that it is because of denial, perhaps by the physician who does not want to acknowledge that he or she is not able to cure the patient and may not feel comfortable having this difficult conversation with the patient and family, or perhaps because the patients and families are in denial themselves.

Unfortunately, but all too frequently, patients who could benefit from palliative care or hospice are not given the opportunity to choose this for themselves. This also means that they are not given the opportunity to have those final conversations or engage in those rituals that may help them to find a deeper spiritual healing and reconciliation. The failure to make referrals in a timely fashion reflects a fear that doing so may contribute to the patient's decline. Sadly, such avoidance only confirms this fear, as those referrals often get postponed until denial is no longer possible, at which point the patient's death confirms the false belief that choosing a palliative approach is synonymous with "giving up" or "choosing death."

This misunderstanding contributes to the false belief that palliative care is contrary to the teachings of Judaism. In fact, Jewish tradition advocates for a compassionate response to those who are suffering and dying, in order to ensure the dignity of the person and remove barriers to the soul's departure from the failing body in those situations where the death of the body is inevitable. Like many Jewish laws, the overarching principle is first gleaned through early rabbinic texts through stories that illustrate this value, and then later, it is codified through rabbinic law.

Jewish Texts

The Talmudic (William Davidson Talmud) text of Avodah Zarah 18a illustrates this perspective by recounting the story of Rabbi Hanina ben Teradyon, who was condemned to death, wrapped in a Torah scroll, and set on fire. His executioners had stuffed his mouth with tufts of wool wet with water, "so that his soul would not leave his body quickly"; however, when an executioner asked if he would be granted Eternal Life in the World to Come by removing the wool from his mouth, Rabbi Hanina replied yes, an affirmation that was later confirmed by a Divine Voice.

From this text, one can see the sacred merit of those who remove barriers to death and suffering for those who are dying. Of course, the previous story may illustrate the principle of removing barriers and decreasing the suffering of an inevitable death, but one might argue that it does not describe a situation where a person is dying through natural causes, such as illness. The Talmudic text of Ketubot 104a depicts a famous story that provides further guidance on the issue of palliative care:

> On the day that Rabbi died, the Sages decreed a fast, and begged for mercy. . . . The maidservant of Rabbi ascended to the roof and said: "The upper worlds are requesting Rabbi and the lower worlds are requesting Rabbi. May it be the Will of G!d that the lower worlds impose their will upon the upper." When she saw how many times he would enter the bathroom and remove phylacteries and put them on and how he was suffering, she said: May it be the Will of G!d that the upper worlds impose their will upon the lower worlds. And the Sages would not be silent from begging for mercy. So she took a jug and threw it from the roof to the ground. The Sages were silent from begging for mercy and Rabbi died.

This story illustrates the natural desire of those close to the person who is dying to wish to prolong that person's life. It also shows the value of doing so, for a time, until the suffering became too great. However, when death is imminent (the timing of a jug thrown to the ground is interpreted by rabbinic tradition to describe the last moments of a person's life), then rabbinic tradition understood the maid's actions of removing the barriers (the begging for mercy) so that the rabbi was able to pass away peacefully.

This rabbinic text contains an important theological understanding, contained in the maid's prayer: "The upper worlds are requesting Rabbi and the lower worlds are requesting Rabbi." When we remove obstacles to a person's dying, we are honoring the "request" of "the upper world." Indeed, one might conclude that a refusal to consider palliative care, and rather to engage in unnecessarily painful, life-prolonging care and medical treatment, is actually creating obstacles to G!d's Will being fulfilled.

This principle was further confirmed by Rabbi Moshe Isserles's commentary on the authoritative halachic (Jewish legal) medieval compendium of the Shulchan Aruch, where he stated that, although it is forbidden to take measures to "hasten one's death," one may "remove obstacles that delay the soul's departure."

This nuance is important, because it highlights the sanctity that rests in the space in between. If we hasten one's death, we will miss out on the important moments that are part of the dying process. For anyone who has worked with those who are dying or accompanied them through this final chapter of one's life on earth, they can attest that this process can be truly holy and healing. Judaism, like most religious traditions, contains sacred rituals, such as the *vidui* or final confessional, which enables patients to connect with family, friends, and G!d, to seek forgiveness and make amends.

When the medical world seeks to prolong a person's dying process through the use of technology and machines, people not only suffer to such an extent that they need to be medicated, they are generally unable to engage in the dying process in an intentional manner. The result is that people are not able to truly live those final moments and engage in those rituals that enable confession, reconciliation, forgiveness, and atonement, and loved ones are robbed of those conversations and connections that are so precious and can be so important for their own grieving and healing process.

The Healing That Palliative Care Provides

Palliative care provides support, care, and comfort measures in ways that often prolong a person's life by improving their quality of life but does not do so in a way that prolongs their suffering or cuts them off from those whom they love. Indeed, the interdisciplinary, whole-person care process facilitates a deep healing of heart, mind, and spirit. Chaplains are often integrated into the care process in ways that the traditional medical model does not, and in so doing, patients and their families have an opportunity to experience pastoral support and healing that they may have been lacking.

In fact, this time is so important and sacred that in the Babylonian Talmud Bava Metzia 87a, it is stated that the biblical patriarch Jacob asked G!d to create illness before death so that children and families can come together at the patient's bedside. Those final conversations are truly sacred, and the palliative care team is specially trained to help facilitate them and to ensure that patients' symptoms are palliated so that they are able to be as present as possible to their loved ones.

In an increasingly secular world, this spiritual component of palliative care is particularly vital. In Hebrew, the word *keruv* means closeness or intimacy and refers to the importance of outreach to those individuals who might feel disenfranchised by organized religion. When people's spiritual needs and concerns are addressed by a chaplain as part of the interdisciplinary palliative or hospice team, the resulting potential healing is profound. Thus, palliative care is now needed more than ever from a spiritual level.

Finally, palliative care plays a crucial role in prevention. Contemporary research demonstrates the risks and complications of unresolved grief and trauma after a loved one's prolonged illness or death (Guldin et al., 2017; Vranceanu, 2019). Without a whole-person interdisciplinary palliative care approach, loved ones frequently suffer posttraumatic stress disorder from watching their loved one suffer. The palliation of symptoms, spiritual support, and meaning making that is possible with palliative care significantly diminishes the risks to the caregiver and improves the quality of life for the patient (Wright et al., 2008).

Contemporary Orthodox scholars such as the modern Orthodox legal scholar Rabbi Moshe Feinstein have reaffirmed Rabbi Isserles's affirmation of the importance of removing obstacles to the dying process. Rabbi Feinstein, in seeking a Jewish answer for the question of palliative care, builds on the Shulchan Aruch law of the middle ages and stated that for "those individuals whom the physicians recognize cannot be cured . . . but could receive medications to extend their lives, in which they would suffer, should not be given such medications" (Feinstein, 1985). This understanding supports the Jewish understanding of the critical importance of palliative care.

The Subjective and Objective Elements of the Dying Experience

The experience of suffering is a defining criterion that would prompt one to consider palliative care, according to both early Talmudic texts and contemporary rabbinic scholars. Despite the fundamental Jewish emphasis on life and the importance of saving a life, which trumps all other legal obligations, rabbinic scholars recognize the importance of palliative care and ensuring that unnecessary suffering not be prolonged. However, the definition of suffering is somewhat subjective.

Dr. Viktor E. Frankl stated that "suffering ceases to be suffering at the moment it finds a meaning, such as the meaning of a sacrifice" (Frankl, 2006). Thus, an important criterion when assessing someone's experience of suffering is their ability to find meaning in their experience, which requires a degree of consciousness. This is yet another reason the incorporation of pastoral care and counseling into a person's care plan is so crucial.

Given the potential subjectivity and variability of a person's experience of suffering, rabbinic tradition has sought to apply a more objective measure to determine the criteria by which "the will of the upper world" – which is to say a person's dying process – should be honored.

In the same way as palliative care can serve as a bridge on the continuum of care between the traditional medical model and hospice, so too does Jewish law seek to identify different approaches to treatment depending on the severity of one's illness. In general, there are two stages of death and dying, the first of which is more subjective than the second.

The first category in Jewish law is called *treifah*, which can be translated as fatal "defects" and refers to those illnesses where one has a reasonable life expectancy of one year or less and for which there is no cure available, while rabbinic literature uses a second Hebrew term, *goses*, to refer to the individual who is actively dying. This stage is generally applied to the last three days of a patient's life (Schostak, 2000).

Both categories warrant a palliative approach; however, the urgency increases as the individual's illness progresses to the state of *goses*. According to Jewish tradition, this state is recognizable by labored breathing. Jewish law mandates a compassionate response where one does not prolong the suffering of a patient in either stage. However, it is also important that one not hasten this time period, as it has its own sanctity.

It may seem like a fine line between "not prolonging" and "not hastening"; however, within this distinction, the deeper theological tenet can be discerned: namely the importance of acting with compassion against suffering while also honoring and preserving life. The subtleties can be seen in the Talmudic statement from Shabbat 151b: "Whoever closes the eyes (of a *goses*) at the moment of death is a murderer." This seems like a very harsh statement that goes against much of the other rabbinic texts that speak to the importance of removing obstacles from one who is dying in order not to prolong the suffering.

The great French medieval commentator Rashi explains that the act of closing the eyes of one who is dying is a reference to the prohibition against hastening death, because "in such a state, even the slightest movement can hasten his death." The authoritative Orthodox legal scholar for our own generation, Rabbi Moshe Feinstein, further clarified: "Touching does not refer to basic care needs such as cleansing and providing liquids by mouth to overcome dryness. [Rather] routine hospital procedures, such as drawing blood or even taking temperature, have no place in the final hours of a patient's life."

Ultimately, decisions regarding end-of-life care require reverence for the sacred Breath of Life that was breathed into the patient and that will be breathed through the patient until it is no longer meant to be so. Hastening or prolonging this Breath is not in our hands to do. Our role is to steward and remove obstacles – be it obstacles to living, which can be called curative care, or obstacles to dying, which can be called palliative care. To allow Breath to flow as it is meant to flow is the ultimate act of reverent witnessing.

Frequently, the argument for palliative care is made based upon compassion. And certainly, compassion should be central to any care decision. But compassion is not enough, as can be seen in the following exhortation by Sefer Hasidim: "Even if a dying patient is suffering from terrible pain and asks someone to kill him, the patient may not be touched. Additionally, a patient who is dying and asks to be moved to another place so he can die there, may not be moved" (Sefer Hasidim 723, from Judah & Finkel, 1997).

If compassion were the sole criteria, one might feel compelled to try to hasten a patient's death in order to reduce his or her suffering. Compassion must be mediated by reverence, and it is in this delicate balance that palliative care is able to dwell. For example, Rabbi Moshe Isserles explains that in the case of someone who has begun the dying process, has become what one might call a *goses*, and is being delayed in his dying process due to the noise made by a woodchopper chopping wood, one is permitted to ask the woodchopper to stop in order to allow the patient to die (Shulchan Aruch Yoreh Deah 339:1).

Reverence for life also requires reverence for its transition points, where the soul journeys from this world into the next. This process is not one to be undertaken lightly, and, indeed, the rabbis recognized its own sanctity. To interfere in this process, or even postpone it, is actually forbidden by many rabbinic authorities, such as Rabbi Solomon Eger in his commentary on Shulchan Aruch, Yoreh Deah 339:1, where he states, "it is forbidden to hinder the departure of the soul by the use of medicines." One might understand many of the modern "aggressive forms of medical intervention" as functioning as a "hindrance" to the departure of the soul.

This recognition that part of reverence includes an acceptance of our mortality can be seen in the Talmud Ketubot 77b, which describes how, when Rabbi Joshua ben Levi, who was known for his great compassion toward those who were sick, was himself about to die, the Angel of Death was instructed, "Go and carry out his wish." As he was journeying toward the heavenly realm, he asked if he could see his place in Paradise before he died and if he could hold the sword of the Angel of Death. As he was granted his wish, he jumped in and refused to return the sword, hoping that this might avert the death of others. G!d said, "Return it to him, for it is required by My mortals."

Ultimately, the delicate balance between curative care, palliative care, and hospice can be found in this tension, whereby compassion must be mediated by reverence for the Breath of Life. Doctors, caregivers, and patients alike must both steward life as best they can and gracefully accept the mortality of the body, which is an inevitable consequence of the life that was given to us in this world.

As the Talmud teaches that the presence of G!d hovers over the bedside of one who is ill, it is considered disrespectful to leave the presence of one who is dying. Indeed, it is encouraged that one wait twenty minutes after a person has passed before the body be moved, as a sign of respect for the soul that is leaving this world to the next, recognizing that no obstacles should impede this journey (Feinstein, 1985).[1]

When the soul finally leaves the body, Jewish law mandates that those present recite a blessing acknowledging G!d as "Dayan Haemet" – the true judge, or the judge of Truth. This prayer encourages an acceptance that the individual's death is part of G!d's will. It is because of this understanding that the removal of obstacles to the patient's death, as palliative care does, is an expression of reverence and faith in G!d's will.

Conclusion

Thus, in conclusion, Jewish tradition affirms the sacred mission of palliative care as a means of caring for patients whose suffering and medical needs are not well addressed by the traditional medical model. The whole-person interdisciplinary approach reflects Jewish beliefs and teachings and ensures a compassionate and reverent approach to end-of-life care.

The traditional Hebrew prayer for healing, the "Misheberach," asks G!d for a *"refuah shleimah, refuat hanefesh u'refuat haguf,"* which is to say, a full and complete healing of body and spirit. When healing of the body is no longer possible, it is still customary to pray this prayer, as the healing of the spirit that is made possible at the bedside of one who is ill is even more crucial. As the soul prepares to leave this world and the body it has been given, it is a sacred time. G!d's presence hovers over the bedside. The way we care for the sick and the dying is one of the most sacred and spiritual acts we can provide. Palliative care provides a method through which medical care and spiritual care can be integrated and, in so doing, enables the field of medicine to actualize the beliefs that are at the heart of Judaism.

The great medieval rabbi, philosopher, legal scholar, and doctor Maimonides is said to have written the following prayer, and while scholars debate the authorship of the prayer, it reflects the humility, faith, reverence, and compassion that Judaism understands to be the mission of medicine. May its humility and reverence serve as a reminder to all people, regardless of faith or tradition, of the importance of always learning, growing, and seeking to improve our understanding and ability to care for one another, "watching over the life and death" of our fellow human beings, for, indeed, in so doing, we partner with G!d in tending to the sparks of life that have been implanted within each person.

> Almighty God, Thou has created the human body with infinite wisdom. Ten thousand times ten thousand organs hast Thou combined in it that act unceasingly and harmoniously to preserve the whole in all its beauty the body which is the envelope of the immortal soul. They are ever acting in perfect order, agreement and accord. Yet, when the frailty of matter or the unbridling of passions deranges this order or interrupts this accord, then forces clash and the body crumbles into the primal dust from which it came. Thou sendest to man diseases as beneficent messengers to foretell approaching danger and to urge him to avert it.

Thou has blest Thine earth, Thy rivers and Thy mountains with healing substances; they enable Thy creatures to alleviate their sufferings and to heal their illnesses. Thou hast endowed man with the wisdom to relieve the suffering of his brother, to recognize his disorders, to extract the healing substances, to discover their powers and to prepare and to apply them to suit every ill. In Thine Eternal Providence Thou hast chosen me to watch over the life and health of Thy creatures. I am now about to apply myself to the duties of my profession. Support me, Almighty God, in these great labors that they may benefit mankind, for without Thy help not even the least thing will succeed.

Inspire me with love for my art and for Thy creatures. Do not allow thirst for profit, ambition for renown and admiration, to interfere with my profession, for these are the enemies of truth and of love for mankind and they can lead astray in the great task of attending to the welfare of Thy creatures. Preserve the strength of my body and of my soul that they ever be ready to cheerfully help and support rich and poor, good and bad, enemy as well as friend. In the sufferer let me see only the human being. Illumine my mind that it recognize what presents itself and that it may comprehend what is absent or hidden. Let it not fail to see what is visible, but do not permit it to arrogate to itself the power to see what cannot be seen, for delicate and indefinite are the bounds of the great art of caring for the lives and health of Thy creatures. Let me never be absent-minded. May no strange thoughts divert my attention at the bedside of the sick, or disturb my mind in its silent labors, for great and sacred are the thoughtful deliberations required to preserve the lives and health of Thy creatures.

Grant that my patients have confidence in me and my art and follow my directions and my counsel. Remove from their midst all charlatans and the whole host of officious relatives and know-all nurses, cruel people who arrogantly frustrate the wisest purposes of our art and often lead Thy creatures to their death.

Should those who are wiser than I wish to improve and instruct me, let my soul gratefully follow their guidance; for vast is the extent of our art. Should conceited fools, however, censure me, then let love for my profession steel me against them, so that I remain steadfast without regard for age, for reputation, or for honor, because surrender would bring to Thy creatures sickness and death.

Imbue my soul with gentleness and calmness when older colleagues, proud of their age, wish to displace me or to scorn me or disdainfully to teach me. May even this be of advantage to me, for they know many things of which I am ignorant, but let not their arrogance give me pain. For they are old and old age is not master of the passions. I also hope to attain old age upon this earth, before Thee, Almighty God!

Let me be contented in everything except in the great science of my profession. Never allow the thought to arise in me that I have attained to sufficient knowledge, but vouchsafe to me the strength, the leisure and the ambition ever to extend my knowledge. For art is great, but the mind of man is ever expanding.

Almighty God! Thou hast chosen me in Thy mercy to watch over the life and death of Thy creatures. I now apply myself to my profession. Support me in this great task so that it may benefit mankind, for without Thy help not even the least thing will succeed. (Author Unknown, 1917).

Discussion Questions

1. With the many interpretations of the Jewish religious text, how can a palliative care physician approach Jewish patients during the end of life?
2. How can the palliative care physicians and healthcare workers aid the community in end-of-life decision-making?

Note

1. "It is customary to wait 20 minutes before the body is touched or moved" (Feinstein, 1985).

References

Author Unknown. (1917). Maimonides' daily prayer of a physician. Translated by Harry Friedenwald. *Bulletin of the Johns Hopkins Hospital* 28, 260–261.

Eilberg, A. (2001). Caring for the dying and their loved ones. In D. A. Friedman (Ed.), *Jewish Pastoral Care: A Practical Handbook from Traditional & Contemporary Sources*. Woodstock, VT: Jewish Lights.

Feinstein, M. (1985). *Responsa Igrot Moshe, Choshen Mishpat*, Vol. 2. New York: Noble Book Press.

Frankl, V. E. (2006). *Man's Search for Meaning*. Boston: Beacon Press. Originally published in 1946.

Guldin, M. B., Ina Siegismund Kjaersgaard, M., Fenger-Grøn, M., Thorlund Parner, E., Li, J., Prior, A., & Vestergaard, M. (2017). Risk of suicide, deliberate self-harm and psychiatric illness after the loss of a close relative: A nationwide cohort study. *World Psychiatry* 16(2), 193–199.

Judah, B. S., & Finkel, A. Y. (1997). *Sefer Chasidim: The Book of the Pious*. Northvale, NJ: Jason Aronson.

Maimonides. (1168). Commentary on the Mishna, Tractate Nedarim 4:4, s.v., "Hamudar hanaa mechaveiro." Fes, Morocco.

National Palliative Care Research Center. (n.d.). About palliative care. www.npcrc.org/content/15/About-Palliative-Care.aspx.

Schostak, Z. (2000). Precedents for hospice and surrogate decision-making in Jewish law. *Tradition* 34, 40–57.

Vranceanu, A. M. (2019). Can we prevent chronic posttraumatic stress disorder in caregivers of critical care patients? *Journal of Emergency Critical Care Medicine* 3, 2.

Wright, A. A., Zhang, B., Ray, A., Mack, J. W., Trice, E., Balboni, T., . . . Prigerson, H. G. (2008). Associations between end-of-life discussions, patient mental health, medical care near death, and caregiver bereavement adjustment. *Journal of the American Medical Association* 300(14), 1665–1673. doi:10.1001/jama.300.14.1665.

Chapter 5

Palliative Care

A Hindu Perspective

Vidya Viswanath and Seema Rajesh Rao

The principal of autonomy is a reflection of cultural values. Unlike Western cultural values, in Hinduism, duty overrides individual autonomy, and filial duty requires that family members take care of, and make decisions for, one another. This is true for all the various groups associated with the Hindu religion and way of life. Such requisite duty provides dignity for all, but this intercollective allowance for decision-making may inadvertently negate the pursuit of dignity of the patient when viewed through a Western lens. The suffering that comes near the end of life is seen as a penance to atone for past sins, and this acceptance collides with Western beliefs that go to great lengths to avoid pain. Death, when it comes, is not seen as something to invoke grief but as an evolution of the soul, closely connected to moksha, *or spiritual liberation. It is not the opposite of life but the opposite of birth. As in earlier chapters, it is vital that the palliative care teams be aware of the psychosocial and spiritual practices of their patients to enable the transition through death to align closely with cultural values.*

Hinduism

Hinduism is a religion that originated in India and is practiced in the Indian subcontinent and Southeast Asia. It is the third-largest religion, with roots dating back more than 4000 years, between 2300 BCE and 1500 BCE (Basham, 1989). Hinduism has no specific founder and evolved as a synthesis of various regional schools of thought, traditions, and philosophies. Hinduism is henotheistic, believing in one, ultimate, divine essence while at the same time recognizing the existence of various Gods and Goddesses (Alon, Gruenwald, & Singer, 1994).

Hindus believe there are multiple paths to reaching the same God. Scholars often refer to Hinduism as "a way of life" rather than a single organized religion (Thillainathan, 2009). In the absence of set rules and dogmas, various diverse and contradictory beliefs coexist within Hinduism. While engaging in a dialogue with a Hindu, it is important to acknowledge this diversity and elicit the specific beliefs and practices of the individual (Sharma, 1999).

The doctrines of *samsara, karma*, and *moksha* are the key tenets of Hinduism. These tenets can guide an individual's actions and impact how a Hindu lives and faces suffering and death.

Hindus believe in reincarnation or rebirth. *Samsara* is the wheel of life, the continuous cycle of death and rebirth that human beings are caught up in as a consequence of their desires and actions. Hindus believe the body is mortal and perishes on death. The soul is eternal and is reborn in another body. All life forms pass through a series of incarnations, and the moral behavior and spiritual advancement in a previous life determine what form the next incarnation may take.

The action of performing one's duties, in thoughts, words, and deeds, with a sense of attachment, is termed *karma*. It is believed that a person living a good life, performing more good deeds than bad, and leading a devout life will be born into a more fortunate existence, while bad karma will lead to more suffering in the next birth. One cannot escape the consequences of one's karma. Birth and death are considered transitions in the cycle of life. Death is not the opposite of life but the opposite of birth (Sharma, 1999).

Hinduism believes that humans are given many chances to perfect their karma and purify their soul through the process of birth and rebirth and become one with *Paramaatma*. This is termed *moksha*. The ultimate purpose of human life is *moksha*, which emancipates one from the cycle of birth and rebirth.

Palliative Care

Living with serious health-related suffering is one of the toughest transitions in life. Bridging evidence and emotion, the role of palliative care is pivotal in addressing this suffering and alleviating the physical, psychosocial, emotional, and spiritual distress that accompany this suffering, in addition to supporting the caregiver. From the patient's perspective, it means finding tranquility amid the turmoil and involves living and facing death with dignity. From the caregiver's perspective, it involves fulfilling multiple roles, living in anticipatory grief, and dealing with conflicting thoughts and emotions. Thus, both the patients and the caregivers require continued support to deal with this transition.

For the physician, the practice of palliative care begins with enhancing and preserving patient dignity along the course of the illness until death. This is done by providing adequate symptom control, respecting autonomy, communicating effectively, making ethical decisions, and navigating through end-of-life care and bereavement support for the patient and his or her caregivers. The goal is to ease transitions, keep hope alive in the face of despair, and maintain the delicate balance between holding on and letting go. Along with evidence-based medicine, the philosophy of Hinduism and the plethora of teachings and stories inspire and influence the practice of palliative care in India.

Dignity in Hinduism

Dignity in Self

Hinduism recognizes the inherent dignity of human beings, acknowledging the intrinsic worth of human existence. The Upanishads describe the entire human race as *Amritasya Putrah* (Sons of the Immortal), thereby highlighting the immortality and divinity of the human race. The invisible individual soul or inner self, the *Atma*, dwells in each body. The soul is eternal, divine, and an extension of the Supreme Soul, the *Paramaatma*. Human beings, living things, and Gods are not distinct selves but part of the same entity. Thus, every living being is equal, has an intrinsic worth or basic dignity (Kant, 2005), and should be treated with respect.

The *Rig Veda*, the first of the four Vedas, emphasizes that "No one is inferior or superior; all are brothers; all should strive for the interest of all and progress collectively" (*Rig Veda Mandala 5, Sukta 60, Mantra 5*).

Personal dignity, on the other hand, is the personal sense of worth that is tied to an individual's personal goals and social circumstances. In palliative care, the concept of dignity in addition to ideas of self-respect and self-worth encompasses an umbrella of terms like meaning/purpose in life, autonomy, physical comfort, spiritual comfort, interpersonal connectedness, belongingness, and courage in the face of impending death (Kissane, 2010). The essence of leading a dignified life for a Hindu encompasses all of the previous virtues, albeit a bit differently from the Western concepts.

Living With Dignity

Hinduism upholds the universal oneness of human beings based on the ideologies of *Vasudaiva Kutumbakam*, which considers the "whole world as a family," as we are all extensions of the Supreme Soul. Hindu culture emphasizes that the whole universe is connected and dependent on one another. The entire universe supports and works to sustain mankind. Hindus believe that every human being by birth carries a debt toward the universe – that is, the debt toward ancestors (*pitr*), toward environment (*deva*), toward culture (*rishi*), toward creatures (*bhuta*), and toward fellow beings (*manushya*). The primary obligation of every Hindu is to clear these debts. The purpose and meaning of life in Hinduism is encompassed in living a righteous life and performing the prescribed duties (*dharma*).

In the presence of terminal illness, the inability to fulfill the prescribed responsibilities or roles can be a source of suffering for a Hindu (Thrane, 2010). The essence of personal dignity in Hinduism entails not in asserting one's rights (*Adhikara*) or in fulfilling one's desires, but in the selfless pursuit and fulfillment of one's duties. Many Hindu families gracefully accept caregiving as their own responsibility, as they consider it their moral duty to look after and protect their loved ones. These beliefs impact autonomy and decision-making. Individual autonomy is perceived as isolating (Searight & Gafford, 2005), with healthcare decisions being made by families, especially the senior male member or the eldest son, rather than the patient. The need to protect also results in families colluding to conceal the diagnosis, prognosis, and treatment information from the patient (Atesci et al., 2004). These concepts differ greatly from those in Western culture, and this variation needs to be respected while dealing with Hindu patients.

Dignity in Suffering

The concepts of karma, rebirth, and *moksha* guide a Hindu's response to suffering. All forms of suffering, physical and mental, are considered to be atonement for inappropriate actions in the past life. Suffering is not viewed as punishment but as essential for resolving karmic issues. Working through these issues is essential in order to have a better life and move toward salvation or *moksha*. Patients and caregivers understand that what they are currently going through is a result of their past karma, and as something they have no control over. They also realize that they can control how they cope with the suffering today, and their action today will have an impact on their future births. This concept of karma answers the toughest question in palliative care: "Why me?" Many times, these answers come from conversations with patients and caregivers without even spelling out the question (Simha, Noble, & Chaturvedi, 2013). For a Hindu, suffering is not random, and pain and suffering are perceived as pathways to spiritual progress and to be borne with fortitude (Simha et al., 2013). To quote Rabindranath Tagore, "Let me not beg for the stilling of my pain but for the heart to conquer it." Hindu patients may choose to endure suffering as a form of penance for past sins, fast or refrain from eating certain types of food, and participate in religious ceremonies or rituals to atone for sins in the past life. They may refuse opioids and pain medications, believing that pain needs to be endured. Some others believe that prayer and rituals alone can cure disease. Acknowledging that beliefs, superstition, and stigma surrounding disease are commonplace, one needs to be both gentle and firm to balance beneficence and autonomy while continuing to care for patients and families. This is why effective communication is the core of palliative care.

Communication

The Hindu equivalent of the Hippocratic oath from the Caraka Samhita 111.8.7 upholds truth telling and confidentiality and respects posthumous arrangements and proxy decision-making in the family (Sharma, 1999). Communicating with equipoise and empathy is the foundation of the professional relationship, which is inclusive of the person and family without being intrusive. The prime focus in the conversation is usually on "today": what troubles the patient most and how best the distress can be alleviated. It is about providing comfort in the present without guilt from the past and worry about the future.

The message from the Divine Song, the Bhagavad Gita, spells this out: "Do not weep for the past; do not worry for the future, concentrate on your present."

As simple as this may seem, it can be really difficult in practice. Conveying this is a crucial part of consultation in the practice of palliative care. This is again where the priceless teachings from the Bhagavad Gita, the epitome of the most powerful communication skills, are invaluable. This is set in the battlefield, and the prime mover, Lord Krishna, does not pick up a weapon. He is the warrior's charioteer. The power of Lord Krishna's listening, his role as a charioteer in guiding the warrior, is akin to the principles of good communication practice like the "Ask–Tell–Ask" approach recommended in practice. This helps to empower patients to make their decisions and aids them in finding the best possible solutions in the given circumstance.

Ethical Dilemmas

Ethical dilemmas are commonplace, and training in palliative care reiterates that it is the intention behind the action, not the fruit of the action, that counts. The Holy Gita defines a true worker or a karma yogi as one whose concern is with the action alone, not the results, and one whose motive is not gaining a specific reward for a particular deed. Also, in palliative care, the patient is not abandoned or asked to go home because of lack of curative therapy or predetermined outcome. The best possible is done to relieve suffering and provide comfort until the very end, like the true worker or karma yogi. The true worker also does not sit back quoting inaction. The action of today becomes the destiny of tomorrow. Man can change his destiny not by wishing but by working for it. Being compassionate toward those suffering is commendable, but a true karma yogi has to translate the thought into action. As Dr. Robert Twycross, a pioneer in palliative care, rightly says, it is the anger in compassion that is needed to practice and build awareness in palliative care.

Shared Decision-Making

The anger in compassion could well be the catalyst for improving access to palliative care, but the way to break barriers and integrate palliative care is only by building bridges. Here, the wisdom to discern, the alertness to judge situations, and the ability to persevere with single-minded dedication are needed. Growing up with the Hindu principles of assimilation, plurality, and acceptance makes it easy to work with multidisciplinary teams and alongside caregivers. During tough times, the stories of wisdom and valor that have percolated down generations of Hindus through the Holy Epics like the *Ramayana* and the *Mahabharata* can be inspiring. It is often said that Hinduism is about rituals, but practicing some of these can inculcate discipline and provide solace. For practicing Hindus, worshipping the image of a deity that personifies

God is a way of connecting with the Supreme Being. Some patients do find it comforting to keep an image of their favorite deity with them. Little *poojas* (ritualized worship) being arranged at the behest of patients, and weddings being solemnized at the hospice go a long way in respecting the personhood of the patients and their families. Quite akin to a temple, hospice is a place where one tries to find peace amidst the turmoil (Viswanath, 2016).

Fulfilling Desires

Toward the end, as palliative care physicians, prioritizing unfinished businesses and focusing on patient's wishes and trying to fulfill them is a constant endeavor. The principle of *moksha* in Hinduism describes this beautifully. It is said that "When life ends and desire remains, it is death and when desire ends and life remains, it is *moksha*." The pursuit of spiritual liberation – that is, self-awareness and self-realization, enlightenment, unity with the Paramaatma, and liberation from the cycle of death and rebirth – is the main purpose in life of every Hindu. The Bhagavad Gita (2:22) states, "As a man casts off his worn-out garments and takes on new ones, so does the embodied self cast away worn-out bodies and enters other new."

This is usually how caregivers go through the cycle of grief and reach acceptance, considering death as an evolution of the soul. This belief that the soul is only a temporary occupant of the body also helps some patients to stoically accept death without fear.

Preserving Dignity in Death

Hinduism considers death a natural and inevitable culmination of life. Hindu scriptures talk about preparing for death, as one enters old age, by giving up worldly life (*vanaprastha*) transitioning into *sanyasa*, or complete renunciation and spiritual pursuit (age 50 onward). One is expected to prepare for a good death throughout life by adhering to and fulfilling one's duties, setting affairs in order, seeking forgiveness, and resolving conflicts. Hindus believe in neither prolonging life nor in hastening death, as it interferes with karmic debt. Hindus believe that death should occur at the right age, at the right time, at the right place. Most Hindus prefer death at home surrounded by family and friends. The thoughts at the time of death determine posthumous destiny, and thoughts of God while dying ensure liberation (Sharma, 1999). A powerful treatise to end-of-life care in Hinduism is the recitation of the Srimad Bhagavatham to King Parikshit when he had only seven days to live. Even today, listening to this discourse is considered the route to salvation.

Response to Loss and Bereavement

The silver hour and bereavement care in palliative care have parallel concerns and rituals in Hinduism, too. Fasting before death, having family around and being conscious of the surroundings, listening to chants being whispered in the ears or played in the background are practiced in the hope of having a good death. The rituals that follow for the next year can keep the family together and prevent complicated grief. In India, it is the extended family and the community, their interconnectedness and interdependence, that absorb the responsibility of taking care of the bereaved to a large extent.

Maintaining Faith and Equipoise

Between holding on and letting go, the practice of palliative care is synonymous with balance. Equipoise both in its practice and within oneself should be maintained. The emphasis in Hinduism is on awakening the soul, having faith in oneself, and drawing into one's own *Shakti* or spiritual force. To achieve the ability to make the mind turn inward to experience self, one has to develop a mental equipoise. A classic analogy is the dancing posture of Lord Shiva in the form of Nataraja. This divine dance, the Thandavam, depicts the flux in the world symbolizing creation and destruction; birth and death transition majestically from the gentle to the violent. Seemingly in conflict, the Lord still maintains rhythm and harmony and combines pulsating energy with perfect balance in this posture where he is called Nataraja.

Amid the multitasking, given the palliative care setting in India, finding this equilibrium is important, and self-care must not be forgotten. This is where India's gift to the world – yoga – is a powerful way to control both the body and mind (Sharma, 1999). Mindfulness, introspection, and reflection along the practice of palliative care actually fill one with gratitude and bring one closer to one's own faith.

Discussion Questions

1. How does understanding the bigger picture (culture competency), communicating with respected key leaders (family), and respecting patients' wishes contribute to more compassionate palliative care?
2. What are some of the implications of physicians' mediations in the Hindu community?

References

Alon, I., Gruenwald, I., & Singer, I. (1994). *Concepts of the Other in Near Eastern Religions*, 370–371. Leiden, NL: Brill Academic Press.

Atesci, F. C., Baltalarli, B., Oguzhanoglu, N. K., Karadag, F., Ozdel, O., & Karagoz, N. (2004). Psychiatric morbidity among cancer patients and awareness of illness. *Supportive Care in Cancer* 12(3), 161–167.

Basham, A. L. (1989). The beginnings of religion in South Asia. In K. G. Zysk (Ed.), *The Origins and Development of Classical Hinduism*, 1–20. New York: Oxford University Press.

Kant, I. (1785/2005). Transition from popular moral philosophy to the metaphysics of morals. In L. Denis (Ed.), *Groundwork for the Metaphysic of Morals*. Peterborough, ON: Broadview Press.

Kissane, D., Treese, C., Brietbart, W., McKeen, N., & Chochinov, H. (2010). Ethical, existential, and spiritual issues in palliative care. In H. Chochinov & W. Breaitbard (Eds.), *Handbook of Psychiatry in Palliative Medicine*, 2nd ed., 324–340. New York: Oxford University Press.

Searight, H. R., & Gafford, J. (2005, February). Cultural diversity at the end of life: Issues and guidelines for family physicians. *American Family Physician* 71(3), 515–522.

Sharma, A. (1999). The Hindu tradition: Religious beliefs and healthcare decisions. In *Religious Traditions and Healthcare Decisions: Religious Beliefs and Their Application in Health Care, a Reference Guide*, 1–18. Chicago, IL: Park Ridge Center for the Study of Health, Faith, and Ethics.

Simha, S., Noble, S., & Chaturvedi, S. (2013, May). Spiritual concerns in Hindu cancer patients undergoing palliative care: A qualitative study. *Indian Journal of Palliative Care* 19(2), 99–105. doi:10.4103/0973-1075.116716.

Thillainathan, N. (2009). Rogers to reincarnation: Counseling people of the Hindu faith. *Psychotherapy Australia* 15(4), 51–52.

Thrane, S. (2010). Hindu end of life: Death, dying, suffering, and karma. *Journal of Hospice and Palliative Nursing* 12(6), 337–342,

Viswanath, V. (2016). Hospice – Where peace and turmoil coexist. *Journal of Pain and Palliative Care Pharmacotherapy* 30(1), 53–54. doi:10.3109/15360288.2015.1134750.

Chapter 6

Palliative Care

A Christian Perspective

Mark E. Murphy

The literature shows that those with no tradition of death have a less difficult time coming to terms with the need for palliative care over aggressive measures or death in general. For example, when a poor or terminal prognosis is given, there is no need to close the gaps of karma or wait for the miracle of the universe. There is no reliance on prayer or a deep look into the why of suffering. The reality of death is more factual and yet no less threatening. This group of reflections represents a community of difference, all of whom are all seeking the soul's purpose, the peace of something, and the hope for those they have grown to love and honor throughout their earthly existence. Thus, though they may be less likely to be involved in an ethical consult or dilemma, they do not escape the pain of what it is to be human, to be physiological, and to lose this place in one's self.

The importance of understanding the context of a patient's religion in healthcare has been illustrated in numerous published studies (Balboni et al., 2013; Balboni et al., 2007; Balboni et al., 2010; Chakraborty et al., 2017; Ehman et al., 1999; Johnson et al., 2014; Koenig et al., 1989). For example, a 2001 multicenter study by MacLean et al. showed that two-thirds of all patients felt that physicians should be aware of their religious or spiritual beliefs in the provision of healthcare (Machado, 2007b). Indeed, spiritual and religious aspects of care constitute one of the eight core domains of palliative care (Breitbart, 2014; Kelly & Morrison, 2015).

The Christian religions, founded as an outgrowth of the Second Temple Judaic ministry of Jesus Christ of Nazareth, spread from the humble beginnings of a band of 12 Jewish disciples in the Galilean wilderness to span the entire globe. Today, two millennia after the death of Christ, it is the world's largest religion, with over 2.4 billion followers, or roughly a third of the world's population (Matsa, 2019). The Roman Catholic Church has an estimated 1.3 billion adherents, the various Protestant denominations have an estimated 900 million members, the Eastern Orthodox Churches contain 270 million followers and the Oriental Orthodox Church another 76 million (Adherents, n.d.; Olson et al., 2018; Rhodes, 2015). There are thousands of different Christian denominations among these three large groups (Olson et al., 2018; Religion in America, 2015; Rhodes, 2015). It is therefore impossible, in the pluralistic and heterogeneous Christian community of today's world, to generalize every fine nuance of a Christian approach to palliative care. However, certain guiding principles, rooted in the fundamental teachings of Jesus Christ, can be delineated that can serve as general guidelines for the provision of palliative care for Christian patients. This chapter outlines those fundamental principles and then applies them in describing several issues central to the palliative healthcare discussion. Specifically, discussions are undertaken regarding how current palliative care concepts mesh with the Christian viewpoints on life, death, and the afterlife. The definition of death, the use of advanced directives, the idea of using extraordinary measures to prolong life, euthanasia and physician-assisted suicide, meeting the physical requirements of the terminally ill (nutrition, hydration, pain control, etc.), and miscellaneous other denomination-specific concerns that must be taken into consideration when dealing with individual patients are all discussed.

A Brief History of Christianity

The Christian faiths all trace their existence to the ministry of Jesus Christ of Nazareth, in the Roman provinces of Galilee and Judea. Most authorities place the beginnings of Christ's ministry around the year 28 CE, with his death by crucifixion (and subsequent resurrection) around the year 31 CE (Woodhead, 2004). Christ's ministry was continued after his ascension into heaven by his 12 original disciples, along with other notable converts such as the Apostle Paul. The early Christian church spread throughout the Mediterranean basin, with prominent early Christian ministries in cities such as Antioch, Alexandria, and Rome. These ministries, loosely connected at first, ultimately came to be led by the bishop of Rome, who eventually took the title of pope as the head of the Roman Catholic Church. After years of persecution, Christianity became the official state religion of the Roman Empire in 381 CE (Woodhead, 2004). The Oriental Orthodox Church, a group of adherents based primarily in Armenia, northern Africa, the Middle East, and India, split from the Catholic Church over different viewpoints about the nature of Christ's divinity in 451 CE (Olson et al., 2018; Woodhead, 2004). A schism between the Eastern and Western church factions, largely over papal primacy, led to the division between the Roman Catholic Church and the Eastern Orthodox churches in 1054 (Olson et al., 2018; Rhodes, 2015; Woodhead, 2004). The Protestant Reformation began in 1517 when the German monk Martin Luther published his Ninety-Five Theses. Numerous other Protestant denominations propagated thereafter (Engelhardt & Smith Iltis, 2005; Engelhardt, 2011; Olson et al., 2018; Religion in America, 2015; Rhodes, 2015; Woodhead, 2004).

Although intrinsically heterogeneous, all varieties of the Christian faith have a few unifying principles (Engelhardt, 2011; Habgood, 1985; Jayard et al., 2017; Koenig et al., 2012; Woodhead, 2004). First, they acknowledge Jesus Christ as the Son of God. Moreover, they believe that the miracle of Christ's crucifixion and subsequent resurrection three days later is proof of His divinity. Acceptance of that idea – the concept of belief that Christ, God's only son, died for the sins of all mankind, and that His resurrection is exemplary of the ability of all believers to conquer death through faith – is, to Christians, the sole means of achieving eternal life (justification by faith). As a result, life and death are intrinsically intertwined in Christianity. The universal Christian focus upon the afterlife has an impact on every approach to patients with terminal illnesses, irrespective of the specific denomination. The Christian idea of eternal salvation, with the immortal soul being only a temporary resident of the physical body, affords Christian patients a wholly different perspective on the death of that physical body than an individual who regards this present life as being all there is (Clarfield et al., 2003; Engelhardt & Smith Iltis, 2005; Engelhardt, 2011; Habgood, 1985; Jayard et al., 2017; Koenig et al., 2012; Markwell, 2005; Mathew-Geevarughese et al., 2019; Pauls & Hutchinson, 2008).

The concept that life is inherently sacred – a gift from God – is also an important component of the general Christian perspective on healthcare. Hazel Markwell, writing in the *Lancet* in 2005, made the point that two basic human values – human dignity and the interconnectedness of every individual – ground all others (Markwell, 2005). In that vein, the preservation of basic human dignity and the mandate to engage Christian charity in order to address the needs of the less fortunate should be drivers of much of the decision-making in a Christian approach to healthcare. This approach is exemplified in Christ's message in the Gospel of Matthew (25:40), which states, "insofar as you did this to one of the least of my brothers, you did it to me." The most fundamental expression of this Christian perspective on healthcare resides in the care of those with serious illnesses. It is this perspective that provides the foundation for a Christian approach to palliative care.

Palliative Care: A Christian Overview

The medical specialty of palliative medicine is a relatively new one. Its efforts are often confused with hospice care – and although the goals of the two are often aligned, there are distinctions that must be made between the two.

The first modern hospice facility was St. Christopher's Hospital, founded in London by Dame Cicely Saunders in 1967 as a means of caring for patients with advanced terminal cancer (Clark, 2000). The first US hospice was founded by Florence Wald, the former dean of the Yale School of Nursing, in Branford, Connecticut, in 1974 using Dame Cicely's example (Friedrich, 1999). Today, enrollment and payment systems for hospice vary from country to country. In the United States, hospice is a specific and separate system of care for the terminally ill (Kelley & Morrison, 2015). Formal enrollment in hospice in the United States currently requires an anticipated survival of less than six months and a willingness to forego potentially curative treatments. US Medicare hospice guidelines require the relinquishment of Part A services.

Palliative care, by contrast, is an interdisciplinary specialty focusing on improving the quality of life for patients with serious illnesses and their families. There is no anticipated survival requirement, and patients may continue all life-prolonging and disease-directed treatments (Kelley & Morrison, 2015). Palliative care is an integrated program that involves medicine, social work, nursing, chaplaincy, and other resources as appropriate (Breitbart, 2014; Centeno et al., 2018; EN: Palliative Care, 2004; Kelley & Morrison, 2015). First recognized as a subspecialty by the American Board of Medical Specialties in 2006, palliative medicine requires an additional year of fellowship after completion of a residency in any of eight medical specialties (Centeno et al., 2018; Kelley & Morrison, 2015; The Joint Commission, 2011).

At the present time, palliative medicine is critically underserved as a US medical specialty (Lupu, 2010). There is one palliative care specialist for every 1200 patients with a serious illness in the United States. As a measure of contrast, this compares with one oncologist per every 141 US cancer patients (Kelley & Morrison, 2015).

The Christian approach to palliative care can be illustrated vividly through an examination of the life of Dame Cicely Saunders (Clark, 2000). Dame Cicely was a nurse, social worker, and doctor who was originally an agnostic but who converted to Christianity as an adult. Her strong Christian faith and multidisciplinary background, coupled with her observations as a caregiver for the terminally ill, led her to formulate the idea that dying patients can experience distress from their physical, social, psychological, and spiritual needs. Dame Cicely felt that all of these needs should be directly addressed via a unified team approach in the dying patient. It is from her holistic approach that the modern specialty of palliative medicine has arisen (Breitbart, 2014; Centeno et al., 2018; Clark, 2000; EN: Palliative Care, 2004; Jayard et al., 2017).

Understanding the Christian perspective on life, death, and the afterlife is at the epicenter of any discussion of the Christian approach to palliative care. Christianity, as a faith, centers on the death of Jesus Christ and his subsequent resurrection, victorious over death, three days later. The pain and suffering of Christ in many ways is mirrored by the pain and suffering of the dying individual. His resurrection is the ultimate resolution of the Christian paradox: proof that faith can conquer death and render each of us immortal. The inherent sanctity of life underscores traditional Christian prohibitions against suicide. However, that same understanding of life's precious nature affords the Christian patient the need to die with dignity and encourages avoidance of the excessive use of heroic measures in an all-consuming pursuit of prolonging one's corporeal existence (Engelhardt & Smith Iltis, 2005; Jayard et al., 2017). The Christian approach to palliative care is therefore a balancing act, incorporating elements of controlling the various physical, social, psychological, and spiritual forms of distress experienced by patients with serious illnesses while at the same time taking appropriate measures to preserve one's life and well-being (Engelhardt & Smith Iltis, 2005; Habgood, 1985; Markwell, 2005).

Specific Christian Issues Regarding Palliative Care

In the context of the previous discussion, there are philosophical issues that routinely arise in the care of the seriously ill patient. Christian providers will interpret these situations through the prism of their faith (Jayard et al., 2017; Koenig et al., 1989; Koenig et al., 2012). Christian patients and their family members will be similarly guided by their interpretations of scripture and their need to reconcile those perspectives with the clinical situation at hand. It is therefore important, in the context of the provider–patient relationship, to understand those perspectives so that the ultimate needs of the patient and family are met to the mutual satisfaction of all parties involved. Some of the more controversial areas involve the use of advanced directives and the definition of death, the use and misuse of heroic measures in defining the limits of care, methods of meeting the physical needs of the dying patient (pain control, nutrition, and hydration), and the use of euthanasia or physician-assisted suicide. Other denomination-specific issues may need to be considered as well (Engelhardt & Smith Iltis, 2005; Koenig et al., 2012; Markwell, 2005; Mathew-Geevarughese et al., 2019; Olson et al., 2018).

Religious Implications of the Definition of Death

The recent Jahi McMath case in Oakland, California, illustrates some of the controversies regarding the definition of death (Schmidt, 2018). McMath was 13 years old in 2013 when a routine tonsillectomy resulted in significant bleeding, ultimately leading to cardiopulmonary arrest. After resuscitation, she was determined to have sustained significant anoxic brain injury. Two days after the arrest, she was determined to be brain dead. Doctors urged her family to take her off life support and donate her organs. However, the life-support devices that sustained her allowed Jahi's heart to continue beating and her lungs to continue breathing. Her Christian parents insisted that she was still alive and fought to keep her on life support. They eventually moved her to New Jersey, one of a few states where state law allows families to reject the concept of brain death because of religious beliefs. Jahi McMath satisfied all legal criteria for brain death in 2013 and was issued a California death certificate in December of that year. After her transfer to New Jersey, her body was maintained on life support until 2018, when she died a second time of a complication of liver failure and had the unique distinction of having a second death certificate issued, four years after the first, in another state (Burkle et al., 2014; Murphy, 2014; Schmidt, 2018).

The plight of Jahi McMath renewed a discussion about what truly constitutes death. Historically, the cessation of cardiopulmonary function defined the death of a person. Advances in critical care support in the 1960s resulted in a reassessment of this position. A physician-led committee from Harvard published a 1968 paper concluding that patients who meet criteria for a certain type of severe brain injury may be pronounced dead before cardiopulmonary function ceases (A Definition, 1968). This concept ultimately led to the 1981 publication of *Defining Death: Medical, Legal and Ethical Issues in the Determination of Death* by the President's Commission for the Study of Ethical Problems in Medicine, which proposed a uniform statute for determining death by either irreversible cessation of circulatory and respiratory functions or irreversible cessations of all functions of the brain, including the brainstem (President's Commission, 1981). These criteria, endorsed by both the American Medical Association and the American Bar Association, were subsequently adopted in all 50 states as the Universal Determination of Death Act (UDDA) (Burkle et al., 2014). A multidisciplinary task force established similar criteria for pediatric brain death nearly 30 years ago (Machado, 2007b). In 2008, the President's Council on Bioethics refined the concept of brain death as an organism's inability to commerce with the external environment as demonstrated by the absence of spontaneous breathing, which is to be considered the organism's fundamental drive to exist (Burkle et al., 2014). Therefore, the concept of brain death as the death of a person has been perpetuated in both the medical and legal communities for nearly 50 years.

Most Christian denominations have accepted the concept of brain death constituting the death of a person (Setta & Shemie, 2015). For example, the Pontifical Academy of Sciences has declared that brain death is not a synonym for death, does not imply death, or is not equal to death, but "is" death (Battro et al., 2008). However, this is not without some degree of controversy. Some have argued that the concept of brain death is merely a vehicle used to facilitate organ donation (Khushf, 2010; Kumar, 2016; Machado, 2007a). Even the scientific underpinnings of the concept have come under scrutiny in the medical literature (Verheijde et al., 2018), lending scientific credence to those who might challenge the UDDA idea of brain death. Sensitivity to these concerns needs to be at the epicenter of any end-of-life counseling of family members of the critically ill.

The Jahi McMath case illustrates a particular end-of-life conundrum sometimes encountered by healthcare professionals. Numerous studies have demonstrated the enhanced importance of religion and spirituality in the medical decision-making process (Balboni et al., 2013; Balboni et al., 2007; Balboni et al., 2010; Curlin et al., 2006; Johnson et al., 2014; Maclean et al., 2003). Despite the near-universal medico-legal uniformity of the guidelines determining death via the UDDA (Burkle, 2014), certain fundamentalist sects, citing the possibility of a miracle, may refuse to allow discontinuation of supportive measures even after a formal declaration of brain death (Chakraborty et al., 2017; Christian Evangelicals, 2009; Rhodes, 2015; Setta & Shemie, 2015). Healthcare providers should always be sensitive to these issues in guiding patients and their families in their decision-making process during a life-threatening illness.

Advanced Directives and the Use and Misuse of Heroic Measures

The plethora of life-prolonging and life-sustaining options currently available have made the end-of-life decision-making process substantially more complex. Families are often asked whether cardiopulmonary resuscitation should be engaged in the event of cardiopulmonary arrest in discussions about do not resuscitate (DNR) orders (Wijmen et al., 2014). The prospect of intubation and mechanical ventilation must be discussed, as well as the potential use of medications to support blood pressure (pressors). Dialysis in the event of renal failure is also a consideration. In the case of competent adults, the use of an advanced directive or living will can be very helpful in ensuring a patient's needs and desires are met with regard to end-of-life care, allowing an avoidance of familial conflict. Living wills can cover specific aspects of end-of-life care such as the use of CPR in the event of cardiopulmonary arrest, intubation and ventilation, the use of life-sustaining drugs, and enteral or parenteral nutrition (Butler et al., 2014; Tolle et al., 2016; US Legal, n.d.; Wijmen et al., 2014).

A distinction should be made between a *healthcare power of attorney* (sometimes known as durable power of attorney for healthcare) and a *living will* (Butler et al., 2014). A healthcare power of attorney authorizes a designated individual to make medical decisions for a patient if the patient cannot make medical decisions for himself. A living will specifies, in writing, the wishes of the patient regarding end-of-life care in the event that those wishes cannot be communicated directly. The exact application of such documents in the United States varies from state to state. There is federal law in the United States governing living wills as well. Medical facilities that receive Medicaid and Medicare funding are subject to the federal Patient Self-Determination Act (PSDA), which mandates that those facilities tell patients upon admission about their rights to use an advanced directive. The law does not mandate the provision of an advanced directive or require that people have one but merely serves as an instrument of awareness (Butler et al., 2014; Tolle et al., 2016; US Legal, n.d.; Wijmen et al., 2014).

The Christian ideal of striking an appropriate balance between ordinary and extraordinary measures in the prolongation of life has been a point of discussion in the church since the 16th century (Cronin, 1958). Daniel A. Cronin, in 1958, following on original work by American moralist Gerald Kelly, proposed a set of definitions that could still apply today:

> Ordinary means of preserving life are all medicines, treatments and operations which offer a reasonable hope of benefit for the patient and which can be obtained and used without excessive expense, pain or inconvenience.

> Extraordinary means . . . are all medicines, treatments and operations which cannot be obtained without excessive pain, expense or inconvenience, or which, if used, would not offer a reasonable hope of benefit.
>
> (Cronin, 1958; Markwell, 2005)

The Christian ethos with regard to palliative care is guided by these principles. Its focus is to provide relief to patients with severe illnesses and their family members, allowing the withdrawal of futile treatments and a shift in the treatment focus toward individual patient dignity and comfort. It is not aimed at hastening death or at postponing it but rather accepts the inevitable eventual death of the body as a natural consequence of life on Earth. In doing so, palliative care underscores the inherent sanctity of life as God's supreme creation (Engelhardt & Smith Iltis, 2005; Habgood, 1985; Jayard et al., 2017; Markwell, 2005).

Meeting the Physical Needs of Patients

The palliative care approach to patients with serious illnesses uses an interdisciplinary, team-centered approach to provide for patient needs. The most fundamental needs of most patients center on the basic physical necessities that all human beings have in times of crisis: maintenance of adequate hydration and nutrition and control of physical pain. Although this may not seem like a source for much controversy, these variables nevertheless can become issues of conflict in the terminally ill patient.

Hydration and Nutrition

The various Christian faiths all unify around the concept of the inherent sanctity of life. As such, withdrawal of hydration and/or nutrition, which would inevitably lead to death, is generally not something that most Christians would find acceptable. However, although causing the death of a patient through starvation or dehydration is reprehensible and inconsistent with all Christian teaching, providing food or water to those in the final stages of dying can sometimes cause greater hardship than relief. Those caring for patients in those cases may elect to forego these measures (Jayard et al., 2017; Markwell, 2005; Wolenberg et al., 2013). The Catholic bishops of Pennsylvania issued a detailed statement in 1991, revised in 1999, that specifically addressed this issue and that offered guidance for Christians seeking answers about the use of hydration and nutrition (Nutrition and Hydration, 1999). The bishops' statement specifically approved situations such as the withdrawal of intravenous feeding, feeding by gastrostomy, and similar actions in a terminally ill cancer patient whose death is imminent, since this would mean the prolongation of patient suffering without hope of meaningful recovery. In that statement, this example was used to say that weighing the balance of benefits versus burdens makes it relatively easy to decide that this could fall into the category of extraordinary means and that such feeding procedures need not be initiated or may be discontinued.

The previously cited Jahi McMath situation, which was the source of some controversy, is one example in which a patient was maintained nutritionally even after being declared brain dead. The medical decision-making becomes quite a bit murkier when dealing with chronic neurologic conditions that are not terminal. In the Pennsylvania bishops' statement, distinctions were made between the conditions of *coma, psychiatric pseudocoma*, the *locked-in state*, and the *persistent vegetative state*. All of these conditions are generally felt to be reversible with the exception of the last one. Patients in a persistent vegetative state have an almost zero percent chance of meaningful recovery after persisting in that condition for more than a year (Plum & Posner, 2007). The bishops made the statement that if the supplying of nutrition and hydration is of benefit to the patient and causes no undue burden of pain or suffering or excessive expenditure of resources, then it is our duty to provide that nutrition and hydration. If the burdens have surpassed the benefits, then our obligation has ceased. That being said, the bishops stated that, in times of uncertainty about the nature of a patient's clinical situation, it is desirable that the benefit of the doubt be given to the continued sustenance of the life of the unconscious person (Nutrition and Hydration, 1999).

The well-known Terri Schiavo case bears specific examination here (Caplan, 2015). In 1990, at age 26, Florida resident Schiavo had a cardiac arrest that left her with anoxic brain injury. Initially diagnosed as being in a coma, she was ultimately determined to be in a persistent vegetative state, with little hope for recovery. In 1998, after years of unsuccessful efforts to improve her condition through medication, speech and physical therapy, and even the implantation of an experimental thalamic stimulator, Terri's husband, Michael Schiavo, petitioned the Sixth Circuit Court of Florida to remove her feeding tube on the grounds that Terri had no hope of a meaningful recovery and that she would not have wanted to be maintained in her current state. He was opposed in this effort by Robert and Mary Schindler, Terri's parents. Unfortunately, Terri did not have a living will, so her true wishes could not be definitively known. The ensuing legal battle went on for years. Ultimately, Michael Schiavo's request was granted, and Terri died seven days after the feeding tube was removed in March 2005.

The Terri Schiavo case is illustrative of many of the conundrums surrounding the issue of provision of hydration and nutrition to those in a persistent vegetative state. Patients with this condition rarely recover (Nutrition and Hydration, 1999; Plum & Posner, 2007). Their quality of life is poor (Nutrition and Hydration, 1999; Wijmen et al., 2014). Typically unable to obtain nutrition or hydration by mouth, they instead are critically dependent upon feeding tubes (or, in some cases, intravenous feedings). Patients in a persistent vegetative state are highly susceptible to infections, particularly pneumonia; urinary tract infections; or skin, soft tissue, and bone infections from decubiti (pressure sores). Still, in the absence of an advanced directive, it is often left up to anguished family members to decide what is best for the patient. That sort of decision-making can be quite difficult, often pitting the patient's loved ones against one another, as was seen in the Schiavo case. Unfortunately, baser issues of inheritance, expense, and personal inconvenience on the part of the patient's caregivers may also carry weight in the decision-making process (Nutrition and Hydration, 1999). Once again, the ethical foundation upon which the decisions are made in these cases depends upon what constitutes ordinary versus extraordinary treatment. In every case, the provision of ordinary treatment is expected and, indeed, is mandatory. It is the definition of what is extraordinary that is the crux of the matter. Is the provision of hydration and nutrition to a patient in a persistent vegetative state extraordinary? This is a question that must always be considered on a case-by-case basis, with the provision of the patient's best interests always at the epicenter of the discussion (Wolenberg et al., 2013).

Control of Pain

The issue of pain control is another consideration that must be addressed in the terminally ill. Narcotic pain medication can provide relief from suffering, but it may also suppress respiration and decrease blood pressure – in some cases hastening death. The Christian idea of the inherent sanctity of life underscores the very clear and unequivocal biblical prohibition against suicide (self-murder). Similarly, most Christian denominations do not support euthanasia. So how does a Christian reconcile taboos against hastening a person's death with the need to provide comfort to the suffering? This issue can be theologically resolved by the principle of the double effect. Thomas Aquinas, in his work *Summa Theologica*, outlined this principle by saying that it is morally permissible to undertake an act that has double effects – both good and bad – if the following conditions are met: First, the act must not be intrinsically evil but must be good or at least indifferent. Second, the good effect must be the intended outcome and the evil effect the unintended outcome. Third, the good effect must not be caused by the evil effect. Fourth, the unintended evil effect must not outweigh the good effect (Sulmasy & Pellegrino, 1999). The principle of the double effect was applied specifically to the issue of pain relief at the end of life by Catholic bioethicist Bridget Campion, who concluded that the beneficial effects of using morphine for pain relief at the end of one's life outweighed the potential risks, including hastening of death (Campion, 2015). This same logic was applied by Pope Pius XII as far back as 1957, when he stated that the use of narcotics to relieve pain was acceptable as long as the intent was to relieve pain and suffering – even if their use shortened the patient's life (Markwell, 2005).

The Christian Perspective on Euthanasia and Physician-Assisted Suicide

Euthanasia (the voluntary ending of one's life through the actions of another) and *physician-assisted suicide* (whereby a licensed physician facilitates a person's suicide by providing them with the means, usually pharmacologic, by which the patient ends his or her own life) are controversial topics in today's Christian community (Attig et al., 2005; Chakraborty et al., 2017; Cohen, 2015; Curlin et al., 2005). Biblical admonitions against murder are ubiquitous and consistent, including the Sixth Commandment. If life is God's greatest miracle, then taking one's life can be construed as self-murder and is therefore a sin of the highest order. By that same token, euthanasia, either passive (by withholding life-sustaining treatments from a patient) or active (by acting with the intent of bringing about a patient's early death), have traditionally been universally condemned by the various Christian religions (Cohen, 2015; Curlin et al., 2008; Engelhardt & Smith Iltis, 2005; Markwell, 2005). This perspective is particularly true among Orthodox Christians and Roman Catholics (Chakraborty et al., 2017). However, there has recently been some fragmentation among various Protestant denominations about this issue, with some opposing all euthanasia and physician-assisted suicide, others opposing active euthanasia and accepting passive euthanasia, and others accepting both euthanasia and physician-assisted suicide as choices that can be made by individual patients and their family members (Chakraborty et al., 2017; Cohen, 2015; Curlin et al., 2008; Sharp et al., 2012). The United Church of Christ, for example, supports the right of individual patients to choose the manner of their death, respecting individual conscience and choice – including physician-assisted suicide (United Church of Christ, n.d.). A 2009 study undertaken in Belgium found that Christians who regularly attended church were far less likely to advocate euthanasia (23 percent) than were atheists (67 percent) or doubters (54 percent) (Broeckaert et al., 2009). However, another Belgian study from 2006 showed that hospitals and nursing homes in Roman Catholic healthcare systems were receptive to euthanasia in the terminally ill (83 percent in hospitals and 85 percent in nursing homes), demonstrating that these cases cannot be assumed to have uniform treatment even among the more traditional non-Protestant Christian faiths (Gastmans et al., 2006).

Laws governing euthanasia in Western societies have largely been constructed along the traditional Judeo-Christian viewpoints and historically have not permitted either euthanasia or physician-assisted suicide. However, these laws have been changing in recent years (Broeckaert et al., 2009; Cohen, 2015; Curlin et al., 2008; Ganzini et al., 2000; Gastmans et al., 2006; Gill, 2000; Kaldjian et al., 2004). In the United States, although euthanasia is not legal anywhere, physician-assisted suicide is now legal by state law in nine locations (Colorado, Hawaii, Maine, New Jersey, Oregon, Vermont, and Washington, as well as the District of Columbia) and has been mandated by court ruling in two others (Montana and California) (Quill & Sussman, 2019). Internationally, physician-assisted suicide is legal in Switzerland, Albania, Germany, Japan, Canada, and the Australian state of Victoria (Curlin et al., 2008; Quill & Sussman, 2019). Active human euthanasia is legal in the Netherlands, Belgium, Colombia, Luxembourg, and Canada (Curlin et al., 2008; Quill & Sussman, 2019). The changing legal environment in the areas of euthanasia and physician-assisted suicide likely reflects changes in the both cultural and religious viewpoints on these subjects and will remain a subject of some controversy for Christians in the coming years.

Other Denomination-Specific Issues in Palliative Care

Patients undergoing palliative care seek comfort, solace, and relief from pain in the setting of chronic illness. As a result, the palliative care approach is multidisciplinary, involving members of a team that includes healthcare professionals and spiritual counselors. Although Christians share many common beliefs, there are certain Christian denominations whose beliefs mandate the application of special considerations.

Jehovah's Witnesses are a Christian denomination based in the United States with over 9 million adherents. They expressly believe that the consumption of blood in any form is not consistent with the doctrine of their faith and will not take blood or blood products. They will, however, allow organ transplantation. The late rock performer Prince was a prominent Jehovah's Witness. The concept of extraordinary measures may be extended to blood transfusion in the case of Jehovah's Witnesses, who are opposed to transfusion under any circumstance (Olson et al., 2018; Rhodes, 2015).

Evangelical Christians are a heterogeneous group composed of members of the Southern Baptist, Pentecostal, and other religions who view themselves as traditional or conservative in their approach to scripture. They are biblical literalists who believe that the Bible, as the Word of God, is both scientifically and historically accurate. Firm adherents to the concept of the inherent sanctity of life, they are often bitterly opposed to abortion and physician-assisted suicide. Some are even resistant to palliative sedation, withholding of artificial nutrition or hydration in the terminally ill, and even do not resuscitate orders (Centeno et al., 2018; Chakraborty et al., 2017; King & Bushwick, 1994; Olson et al., 2018). Frequently, they will cite the possibility of miracles, which might render hope to a seemingly hopeless medical situation. Evangelicals at times can be inherently suspicious of hospice care. These concerns need to be taken into account when dealing with any evangelical patient with a chronic and possibly terminal illness (Chakraborty et al., 2017; King & Bushwick, 1994; Olson et al., 2018; Rhodes, 2015).

Summary and Conclusions

The Christian perspective on palliative care is rooted deeply in the fertile soil of the Christian faith's long-standing dedication to the inherent sanctity of life itself. Christianity teaches that the soul is immortal; that death of the body is inevitable; and that every person, first loved by God, is deserving of dignity – even in their final hours upon this Earth. The evolving practice of palliative care medicine, with its multidisciplinary approach to the ease of all forms of suffering, meshes well with this Christian ideal.

Most Christians' reverence for the sanctity of life does not mean that the pursuit of extension of one's corporeal existence should trump all other issues. Although there are thousands of Christian denominations, a few general principles illustrating the typical Christian approach to palliative care can be identified. First, distinctions should be made between the use of ordinary measures to extend life and extraordinary measures. Extraordinary measures that are medically futile may expose patients to unnecessary pain, suffering, and expense without any tangible benefit. Second, while hydration and nutrition should not be withheld from terminally ill patients in order to hasten death, it is reasonable to withhold them from those in the final stages of death if those interventions simply prolong a patient's suffering. The use of narcotics to provide relief from pain in the terminally ill is also desirable, even if the use of said medications shortens the patient's life, as long as the goal is relief of suffering. The provision of nutrition and hydration to patients in a persistent vegetative state needs to be addressed on a case-by-case basis, in accordance with patient and/or family wishes and with the careful guidance of the attendant medical professionals. Third, the use of advanced directives in order to more clearly delineate a patient's wishes when they are in extremis can be helpful in eliminating family strife in critical end-of-life times. Fourth, while most Christian faiths do not support physician-assisted suicide and euthanasia, these topics are in both legal and ethical evolution at present, and there has been some fragmentation of the traditional Christian position in recent years.

When dealing with patients and their families during a critical or life-threatening illness, the value of effective communication cannot be overemphasized. Decisions about the care of the chronically or terminally ill are not simply made in a sterile vacuum of the medical literature but instead in the real-world milieu of the patient's life. Involvement of healthcare professionals, patients and their family members, pastoral care representatives, and other ancillary medical staff can allow the focus to remain on providing patients and their families with optimal relief from suffering during the final, inevitable chapter of a patient's life.

The American-British novelist Henry James, on his deathbed, reportedly said, "So, it has come at last, the distinguished thing. Indeed, a Christian believer's temporal death can be exactly that: a peaceful transition into a higher plane of existence, surrounded by loved ones, without angst or suffering. Under these ideal circumstances, death is not perceived as a defeat, but as the ultimate realization of Christ's plan for all of humanity."

Discussion Questions

1. What role does the author's understanding of dignity play in end-of-life care?
2. Can cultural norms negate religious doctrine?

References

A definition of irreversible coma. (1968). Report of the Ad Hoc Committee of the Harvard Medical School to examine the definition of brain death. *Journal of the American Medical Association* 205(6), 337–340. doi:10.1001/jama.205.6.337.

Adherents.com. (n.d.). *World Religions Religion Statistics Geography Church Statistics*. www.adherents.com/.

Attig, T., et al. (2005). Rational suicide in terminal illness. In K. J. Doka (Ed.), *Living with Grief: Ethical Dilemmas at the End of Life*, 175–197. Washington, DC: Hospice Foundation of America.

Balboni, T. A., et al. (2007). Religiousness and spiritual support among advanced cancer patients and associations with end-of-life treatment preferences and quality of life. *Journal of Clinical Oncology* 25(5), 555–560, doi:10.1200/jco.2006.07.9046.

Balboni, T. A., et al. (2010, January 20). Provision of spiritual care to patients with advanced cancer: Associations with medical care and quality of life near death. *Journal of Clinical Oncology*. www.ncbi.nlm.nih.gov/pmc/articles/PMC2815706/.

Balboni, T. A., et al. (2013). Provision of spiritual support to patients with advanced cancer by religious communities and associations with medical care at the end of life. *JAMA Internal Medicine* 173(12), 1109. doi:10.1001/jamainternmed.2013.903.

Battro, A., et al. (2008). Why the concept of brain death is valid as a definition of death. Statement by the Pontifical Academy of Sciences, Extra Series 31. Vatican City.

Breitbart, W. S. (2014). Principles of palliative care. *Psychosocial Palliative Care*, 3–10. doi:10.1093/med/9780199917402.003.0001.

Broeckaert, B., et al. (2009). Palliative care physicians' religious/world view and attitude towards euthanasia: A quantitative study among Flemish palliative care physicians. *Indian Journal of Palliative Care* 15(1), 41–50. doi:10.4103/0973-1075.53511.

Burkle, C. M., et al. (2014). Why brain death is considered death and why there should be no confusion. *Neurology* 83(16), 1464–1469. doi:10.1212/wnl.0000000000000883.

Butler, M., et al. (2014). Decision aids for advance care planning: An overview of the state of the science. *Annals of Internal Medicine* 161(6), 408. doi:10.7326/m14-0644.

Campion, B. (2015, February). Pain relief at the end of life: An application of the principle of double effect. *Bioethics Matters* 13(2), 1–4.

Caplan, A. (2015, March 31). Ten years after Terri Schiavo, death debates still divide us: Bioethicist. *NBCNews.com*. NBCUniversal News Group. www.nbcnews.com/health/health-news/bioethicist-tk-n333536.

Centeno, C., et al. (2018). White paper for global palliative care advocacy: Recommendations from a PAL-LIFE expert advisory group of the Pontifical Academy for Life. Mary Ann Liebert, Vatican City. www.liebertpub.com/doi/10.1089/jpm.2018.0248.

Chakraborty, R., et al. (2017). A systematic review of religious beliefs about major end-of-life issues in the five major world religions. *Palliative and Supportive Care* 15(5), 609–622. doi:10.1017/s1478951516001061.

Christian Evangelicals. (2009). The challenge for hospice and palliative care. In K. J. Doka, et al. (Ed.), *Living with Grief: Diversity and End-of-Life Care*. Washington, DC: Hospice Foundation of America.

Clarfield, A. M., et al. (2003). Ethical issues in end-of-life geriatric care: The approach of three monotheistic religions: Judaism, Catholicism, and Islam. *Journal of the American Geriatrics Society* 51(8), 1149–1154. doi:10.1046/j.1532-5415.2003.51364.x.

Clark, D. (2000). Cicely Saunders – founder of the hospice movement. *APS Bulletin* 10(4).

Cohen, C. B. (2015). Christian perspectives on assisted suicide and euthanasia. *Physician Assisted Suicide* 334–346. doi:10.4324/9781315811369-27.

Cronin, D. A. (1958). *The Moral Law in Regard to Ordinary and Extraordinary Means of Preserving Life*, 471. Rome: Gregorian University.

Curlin, F. A., et al. (2005, July). Religious characteristics of U.S. physicians: A national survey. *Journal of General Internal Medicine*. www.ncbi.nlm.nih.gov/pmc/articles/PMC1490160/.

Curlin, F. A., et al. (2006). The association of physicians' religious characteristics with their attitudes and self-reported behaviors regarding religion and spirituality in the clinical encounter. *Medical Care* 44(5), 446–453. doi:10.1097/01.mlr.0000207434.12450.ef.

Curlin, F. A., et al. (2008). To die, to sleep: US physicians' religious and other objections to physician-assisted suicide, terminal sedation, and withdrawal of life support. *American Journal of Hospice and Palliative Medicine* 25(2), 112–120. doi:10.1177/1049909107310141.

Ehman, J. W., et al. (1999). Do patients want physicians to inquire about their spiritual or religious beliefs if they become gravely ill? *Archives of Internal Medicine* 159(15), 1803–1806. doi:10.1001/archinte.159.15.1803.

Engelhardt, H. T. (2011). Orthodox Christian bioethics: Some foundational differences from Western Christian bioethics. *Studies in Christian Ethics* 24(4), 487–499. doi:10.1177/0953946811415018.

Engelhardt, H. T., & Smith Iltis, A. (2005). End-of-life: The traditional Christian view. *Lancet* 366(9490), 1045–1049. doi:10.1016/s0140-6736(05)67383-7.

EN: Palliative Care. The Solid Facts. (2004). Edited by D. Guest & I. J. Higginson. *1pdf.Net*, 1pdf.net/en-palliative-care-the-solid-facts_585707bae12e8934407728fe.

Friedrich, M. (1999). Hospice care in the United States: A conversation with Florence S. Wald. *Journal of the American Medical Association* 281(18), 1683–1685. doi:10.1001/jama.281.18.1683.

Ganzini, L., et al. (2000). Physicians' experiences with the Oregon Death with Dignity Act. *New England Journal of Medicine* 342(20), 1538–1538. doi:10.1056/nejm200005183422023.

Gastmans, C., et al. (2006). Prevalence and content of written ethics policies on euthanasia in Catholic healthcare institutions in Belgium (Flanders). *Health Policy* 76(2), 169–178. doi:10.1016/j.healthpol.2005.09.003.

Gill, C. (2000). Health professionals, disability, and assisted suicide: An examination of relevant empirical evidence and reply to Batavia (2000). *Centre for Suicide Prevention*, www.suicideinfo.ca/resource/siecno-20011516/.

Habgood, J. S. (1985). Medical ethics – A Christian view. *Journal of Medical Ethics* 11(1), 12–13. doi:10.1136/jme.11.1.12.

Jayard, S. S., et al. (2017). Healing ministry and palliative care in Christianity. *Indian Journal of Medical Ethics* 2(4). doi:10.20529/ijme.2017.054.

Johnson, J. R., et al. (2014). The association of spiritual care providers' activities with family members' satisfaction with care after a death in the ICU. *Critical Care Medicine* 42(9), 1991–2000. doi:10.1097/ccm.0000000000000412.

The Joint Commission. Advanced Certification for Palliative Care Programs. (2011). www.jointcommission.org/certification/palliative_care.aspx.

Kaldjian, L. C., et al. (2004). Medical house officers' attitudes toward vigorous analgesia, terminal sedation, and physician-assisted suicide. *American Journal of Hospice and Palliative Medicine* 21(5), 381–387. doi:10.1177/104990910402100514.

Kelley, A. S., & Morrison, R. S. (2015). Palliative care for the seriously ill. *New England Journal of Medicine* 373(8), 747–755.

Khushf, G. (2010). A matter of respect: A defense of the dead donor rule and of a 'whole-brain' criterion for determination of death. *Journal of Medicine and Philosophy* 35(3), 330–364. doi:10.1093/jmp/jhq023.

King, D. E., & Bushwick, B. (1994). Beliefs and attitudes of hospital inpatients about faith healing and prayer. *Journal of Family Practice* 39(4), 349–352.

Koenig, H. G., et al. (1989, April). Physician perspectives on the role of religion in the physician–older patient relationship. *Journal of Family Practice*. www.ncbi.nlm.nih.gov/pubmed/2784826.

Koenig, H. G., et al. (2012). *Handbook of Religion and Health*. London: Oxford University Press.

Kumar, L. (2016, April). Brain death and care of the organ donor. *Journal of Anaesthesiology Clinical Pharmacology* 32(2), 146–152. doi:10.4103/0970-9185.168266.

Lupu, D. (2010). Estimate of current hospice and palliative medicine physician workforce shortage. *Journal of Pain and Symptom Management* 40(6), 899–911. doi:10.1016/j.jpainsymman.2010.07.004.

Machado, C. (2007a). Brain death and organ transplantation: Ethical issues. *Brain Death*. New York: Springer, 200–207. doi:10.1007/978-0-387-38977-6_8.

Machado, C. (2007b). Brain death in children. *Brain Death*. New York: Springer, 158–168. doi:10.1007/978-0-387-38977-6_6.

Maclean, C. D., et al. (2003). Patient preference for physician discussion and practice of spirituality. *Journal of General Internal Medicine* 18(1), 38–43. doi:10.1046/j.1525-1497.2003.20403.x.

Markwell, H. (2005). End-of-life: A Catholic view. *Lancet* 366(9491), 1132–1135. doi:10.1016/s0140-6736(05)67425-9.

Mathew-Geevarughese, S. E., et al. (2019). Cultural, religious, and spiritual issues in palliative care. *Primary Care: Clinics in Office Practice*. doi:10.1016/j.pop.2019.05.006.

Matsa, K. E. (2019, June 25). World's largest religion is still Christianity. *Pew Research Center*. www.pewresearch.org/.

Murphy, M. E. (2014, February 2). There's something to be said for dying with dignity. *Savannah Morning News*.

Nutrition and Hydration: Moral Considerations. (1999). pacatholic.org/bishops-statements/nutrition-and-hydration, Accessed June 24, 2019.

Olson, R. E., et al. (2018). *Handbook of Denominations in the United States*. Nashville, TN: Abingdon Press.

Pauls, M., & Hutchinson, R. C. (2008). Protestant bioethics. In P. A. Singer & A. M. Viens (Eds.), *Cambridge Textbook of Bioethics*, 430–435. London: Cambridge University Press. doi:10.1017/cbo9780511545566.063.

Plum, F., & Posner, J. B. (2007). *Plum and Posner's Diagnosis of Stupor and Coma.* New York: Oxford University Press.

President's Commission for the Study of Ethical Problems in Medicine and Biomedical and Behavioral Research. (1981). *Defining Death: Medical, Legal and Ethical Issues in the Determination of Death.* Washington, DC: Government Printing Office.

Quill, T. E., & Sussman, B. (2019). Physician-assisted death. *Hestings Center.* University of Rochester. www.thehastingscenter.org/briefingbook/physician-assisted-death/, Accessed July 1, 2019.

Religion in America: U.S. religious data, demographics and statistics. (2015, May 11). *Pew Research Center's Religion & Public Life Project.* www.pewforum.org/religious-landscape-study/.

Rhodes, R. (2015). *The Complete Guide to Christian Denominations.* Eugene, OR: Harvest House.

Schmidt, S. (2018, June 29). Jahi McMath, the Calif. girl in life-support controversy, is now dead. *Washington Post.*

Setta, S. M., & Shemie, S. D. (2015). An explanation and analysis of how world religions formulate their ethical decisions on withdrawing treatment and determining death. *Philosophy, Ethics, and Humanities in Medicine* 10(1). doi:10.1186/s13010-015-0025-x.

Sharp, S., et al. (2012). Religion and end-of-life treatment preferences: Assessing the effects of religious denomination and beliefs. *Social Forces* 91(1), 275–298. doi:10.1093/sf/sos061.

Sulmasy, D. P., & Pellegrino, E. D. (1999). The rule of double effect: Clearing up the double talk. *Archives of Internal Medicine* 159(6), 545. doi:10.1001/archinte.159.6.545.

Tolle, S. W., et al. (2016). Assessing evidence for physician orders for life-sustaining treatment programs. *Journal of the American Medical Association* 315(22), 2471. doi:10.1001/jama.2016.4024.

United Church of Christ. (n.d.). Faithfully facing dying. www.ucc.org/faithfully_facing_dying, Accessed May 24, 2019.

US Legal, Inc. (n.d.). Uniform Health-Care Decisions Act Law and Legal Definition. *Uniform Health-Care Decisions Act Law and Legal Definition.* definitions.uslegal.com/u/uniform-health-care-decisions-act/.

Verheijde, J. L., et al. (2018). Neuroscience and brain death controversies: The elephant in the room. *Journal of Religion and Health* 57(5), 1745–1763. doi:10.1007/s10943-018-0654-7.

Wijmen, M. P. S. Van, et al. (2014). Continuing or forgoing treatment at the end of life? Preferences of the general public and people with an advance directive. *Journal of Medical Ethics* 41(8), 599–606. doi:10.1136/medethics-2013-101544.

Wolenberg, K M., et al. (2013). Religion and United States physicians' opinions and self-predicted practices concerning artificial nutrition and hydration. *Journal of Religion and Health* 52(4), 1051–1065. doi:10.1007/s10943-013-9740-z.

Woodhead, L. (2004). *Christianity: A Very Short Introduction.* Oxford: Oxford University Press.

Chapter 7

A Nontraditional Spirituality Perspective on Palliative Care and End of Life

Denise C. Thompson

Not everyone belongs to an organized religion, yet palliative care must be given to all. As a believer, how do you counsel the nonbeliever? As a non-believer, how do you counsel a believer? As this author explains, listening compassionately and without judgment can go a long way toward bringing a patient and/or family to peace and acceptance. And sometimes, from non-belief to belief in a higher power.

I had coffee with an atheist the other day. She's actually an atheist chaplain known as a "humanist." I was curious as to how an atheist chaplain ministers to the needs of a patient who is spiritual – which is the opposite of what this chapter addresses: How does a spiritual chaplain minister to the needs of an atheist, who is anything but spiritual?

I used to think being an atheist would be the worst possible existence: live, die, gone. Not to have hope for something beyond this existence is unimaginable for me. For believers, we have hope for life after death, that deathbed goodbyes are a "so long until we meet again." Courtney, my atheist chaplain friend, thinks all of that is claptrap – just a coping mechanism for believers; though having a heart of gold, she respects everyone's belief system and does not judge. She would only ask that we do the same.

As an atheist chaplain, Courtney ministers to the emotional aspect of one's needs, though she respects the spiritual dimension as well, listening compassionately to hopes, dreams, and fears, even praying with believers because – as all chaplains know – it is about the patient, resident, or family and what is important to them; it is not about us.

So what is pastoral care, and what does a chaplain do? Author Emmanuel Lartey (2006) describes pastoral care as an "interaction between two people where the exchange can be explored in the context of care." This is a very succinct way of saying what we do. As chaplains, we reach out to the vulnerable with compassion and create a supportive, trusting presence where patients (or residents or family) can explore what is happening to them and make meaning of it. From this context comes hope. Chaplains minister to people of all faiths or no faith – and it is *their* faith or lack thereof, not ours, that is honored.

Now let's get back to Courtney. Courtney is married and in her 30s. Her atheist belief system gives her life value and purpose. Like most atheists, she looks to science, good stewardship of the Earth's resources, and the pursuit of peace and happiness for all humans as her compass to moral living. Atheists believe that life *is* science, and they embrace its mysteries and wonder. Science begs to be discovered; for atheists, each generation pushes the needle a little further in unlocking some of its secrets. Then they return to the nothingness from which they came, leaving additional discoveries for future generations. For them, this is a good life.

Atheists take offense when well-meaning people try to label them as spiritual by saying things like "The birds of the air are your religion" or "You are spiritual because you commune so easily with nature." Courtney, however, is adamant: "No. I am not spiritual in any way because I do not believe in any kind of spirits or angels or afterlife or nirvana or other-worldly or ethereal. There is no state of mind after death. I believe in science and what is tangible and when I am gone, that's it. I am nothing again."

Courtney says she is not afraid of dying; it is just like going to sleep with nothing to follow. She said she did not exist before she became a "thing" (a tangible being in her mother's womb), so why should she exist afterward?

For Courtney, these are not just words. When she was 32, she had open-heart surgery preceded by the doctor's statement, "I don't know if I can fix this." The fear she felt was not for herself but for her family. "Who will comfort them in their sadness if I die?" Courtney wished a chaplain could sit with them during surgery to offer support and fortitude.

We talked about quality of life and how an atheist's principles might influence end-of-life choices, such as withdrawal of life support. Courtney shared that in her chaplaincy, she experienced that the more religious people were, the harder it was for them to let go, which she thought was ironic. "So, if you really believe in an afterlife, why endure futile suffering and let machines get in the way of your going there?" On the other hand, she believed people who were not spiritual were more likely to face reality and let go.

Courtney mentioned the "Five Wishes" living will. She supports this document because it delves into the emotional and not just the practical aspects of dying. She says "Five Wishes" resonates with her because it encourages people to do what all people really want at end of life, and that is to talk – just talk and have someone listen compassionately without judgment.

Courtney is right in that respect. I had a rich and lovely conversation with a Buddhist suffering from cancer with a life expectancy of six more weeks. She wanted to see a fellow Buddhist but, being a new resident of Savannah, had not yet made connections to that community. She wanted to talk to someone but was adamant it not be a Christian. When the nurse saw me, a Catholic chaplain, heading toward her room, she stopped me. I, on the other hand, just wanted to clarify exactly who the patient wanted to see so I could do my best to find someone.

The Buddhist patient and I were contemporaries and immediately connected. She invited me in and she spoke at length about her family and religion and how she treasured the love and peace they brought her. She said she hoped for eternal tranquility in the next world in whatever form that may be, whether a place or a state of mind. She said she asked not to see a Christian because she feared they would try to convert her, not listen to what was in her heart, and mar the little bit of time she had left. She was not afraid to die, and this death-bed reminiscing and hoping and longing for that in which she believed brought her dignity and spiritual closure on this chapter of her existence.

As the title implies, the remainder of this chapter attends to various forms of nonbelief as well as beliefs of those who consider themselves spiritual but in a nontraditional sense; that is, they seek fulfillment and growth outside of organized religion. Because it would be impossible to include every nontraditional scenario, a range of categories has been selected to illustrate chaplaincy through real-life examples of people facing actual or potential end-of-life situations.

Atheism

Atheists do not believe in the existence of deities. They reject any notion that divine beings exist in any form. When life is over, you cease to be.

Sam, single and in his 40s, was a window washer and professed drug dealer. A loner, he had no religion and no beliefs in higher powers. Unlike Courtney, he had no use for people unless they could serve some tangible need of his own. He was not as comfortable in his own skin as Courtney is in hers. His lack of faith was not a conscious decision, as is Courtney's, who was raised in a religious household. His nonbelief was simply irrelevant, bringing him no solace or sense of purpose.

Sam was scheduled for cancer surgery the next day and was afraid he might die. He had no true friends or family to support him. The whereabouts of his estranged father were unknown. He had no coping mechanism for his fear, no support system.

As I listened compassionately, I noticed a photo of the patient with an enormous snake and asked about it. With that, Sam's solemn, fear-filled face broke into a grin and visibly softened as he spoke of his love for Olivia, his boa constrictor.

He showed me pictures of his snake and told stories of how they sleep in the same bed, how they play hide-and-seek, and the delight he takes in watching her eat – swallowing rodents whole after she torments them.

His stories of Olivia opened him up, expressing his emotions and forgetting his fears for a while. She gave meaning to his life, the only thing that brought him comfort and love. Olivia was his safe haven in a cold world. He worried about her, though, having left her with someone he barely knew to care for her until his return. "He just won't do it right! She must be petrified. I have to survive and get home!"

I ministered to Sam by listening patiently without judgment, encouraging him to verbalize the thing that gave meaning to his life along with hope and fortitude: his relationship with a snake, his loyal companion and one true friend.

Agnosticism

Agnostics neither believe nor disbelieve in God. They simply have no way of knowing if he exists because his existence has never been proven. They remain skeptical unless evidence is uncovered to indicate otherwise.

Cindy adored her husband. They had been married for 39 years, but sadly he died after a courageous and painful battle with cancer. Drew wanted desperately to live regardless of the suffering. He longed to be with Cindy and their children and families, all of whom lived just around the corner. Drew cherished their little home in the cul-de-sac. He loved the backyard birds and built houses, feeders, and baths for them.

When Drew passed away, Cindy was very sad. She did not take solace in any faith tradition because she did not believe there was a God. Admittedly, she did not know for sure but dismissed it, perhaps not wanting to be disappointed. Regardless, it was just not for her.

When I visited with Cindy some months later, she was still in deep mourning. She did not know how to move forward. She was stuck and had no hope of ever being happy again. She was morose, just going through the motions of another day. Rising, walking, eating, and sleeping – all with a heavy heart.

During our visit, I encouraged her to tell stories about her husband, what he liked to do, and what was important to him. She spoke of Drew, a firefighter, and how he loved doing projects on his days off – always building or growing something. He was very skilled and took pleasure in his accomplishments; however, there was one thing that eluded him. He could not get the bluebirds to come to the bluebird house he had built for them. He put it close to the patio, hoping to enjoy their beautiful colors through the window. But they never came, and then he died.

A few weeks after his death, Cindy noticed a bluebird in the bluebird house. It was perched on the birdhouse peering through the window at Cindy. It was strange how the little bird looked at her without flinching, as though he knew her. It was as if he wanted to say, "Don't be afraid. I love you and I am still here."

Cindy opened her heart to new possibilities and allowed herself to imagine, even believe, the bluebird was her husband and ever since pictured the existence of a greater power with a wonderful world where Drew was happy and waiting for her.

Now she smiles when she thinks of the bluebird, pretty sure it was Drew – but whether it was or not, she believes it is a sign that there *is* more after life. The veil of sorrow lifted a little bit on that day and even more in the weeks to come. She allowed herself to enjoy the company of old friends whom she had not called for a long time after his death despite their reaching out to her. She allowed herself to laugh and rejoice in old photos of happier times.

I ministered to Cindy by helping her find meaning in Drew's death and hope in her own life. I gently encouraged her stories, letting the smiles and tears ebb and flow naturally.

Religious Disaffiliation

These are people who leave their faith tradition or spiritual community. It is not clear whether they intend to replace it or to disengage permanently from religious affiliation (Religious Disaffiliation, 2019).

Lucy, a mother of two young children, was a patient in the burn ICU. She and her kids narrowly escaped a raging fire in the middle of the night. Upon smelling the smoke, her nine-year-old daughter screamed "Fire!" and ran out, but her little brother was trapped in his bedroom. Lucy rushed into the fire and rescued him. She was badly burned, but he was worse. He lay in a coma swaddled in bandages across the hall from her room.

At first Lucy would not speak to me, only shrug and cry. She could not bear the image of her five-year-old son fighting for his life. She blamed herself for not getting to him faster, even though she did everything as rapidly as humanly possible, even beating police and fire personnel to the rescue, but she feared it was not enough.

This was not the first tragedy in Lucy's life. She had been badly injured in an Amtrak crash on her 21st birthday. She was going to the city to celebrate with friends. People in her train car screamed and died, and she was sad for them and their families. She became a widow at an early age, losing her first husband to a motor vehicle accident; she remarried, but her second husband died from an illness.

She said God hated her and so she disengaged, living life on her own without him. I listened attentively and quietly, helping the patient with her food as we talked and visiting her at end of shift with bedtime stories. On one occasion, I introduced Lucy to the Book of Job from the Old Testament. Lucy was intrigued by Job and what happened to him and why. He was a devoted servant of God, yet he suffered so much. She was inspired by Job and opened herself up to a relationship with God again.

After a few weeks, her son began to wake up, talk, walk, and heal. Lucy and I gathered around his bed to pray, and as we were assembling his stuffed animals for prayer, Lucy's heart broke when he hung his head and asked in a tiny voice, "Mommy, will we have a home to go to?" Some months later, there was great joy among the staff as he rode out on his toy fire truck on his way to their safe new home.

I ministered to Lucy by allowing her to express her emotions, including her anger at God, and guided her through her guilt and reconciliation. She discovered meaning and hope through a bible story.

Spiritual but Not Religious

This, too, can be widely interpreted, but it generally means people who consider themselves spiritual (open to the existence of powers or beings greater than themselves) but have severed their connection to organized religion (Ammerman, 2013).

Bea was terrified. When I entered her hospital room, she grabbed my hand, looked me in the eyes, and said, "I have a big decision to make tonight." She was tearful and felt all alone, even though family members were with her at her bedside. She had to decide whether to have brain surgery the next morning for a large malignant tumor. She was told there was a 50 percent chance she would die in surgery but a 100 percent chance she would be dead in six weeks if she did not have the procedure.

As Bea spoke, I listened attentively and probed for unspoken emotions that I sensed were there. Consequently, the patient came to realize she was not as afraid of dying as she was of burdening her son and daughter with the unpleasant task of withdrawing life support if it came to that, a very likely scenario. I sensed the family and patient had not talked about what the patient would want in that event, tipped off by her daughter's chanting, "I will support my mom in whatever she wants to do."

I asked the daughter if she shared her mother's fear, and she said no, that if it were to come to that (i.e., change in code status, withdrawal of mechanical ventilation), she would make the decision. She was adamant, however, in telling her mom to do what she wanted, not what she thought the family would want. The reassurance her children would not suffer from such a frightening and sorrowful task gave her peace.

Aware of her spiritual-but-not-religious mindset, I comforted the patient by telling her to breathe the spirit in slowly and deeply and to breathe out any misgivings or negative thoughts, and above all to listen to her own heart and then she would know what to do. By the end of the visit, the patient was no longer sobbing but calm and serene. She had the guidance she needed from her family and chaplain.

The next morning, I found the patient in her room with her son. They were smiling broadly. Her son said his mom decided to forego the surgery. Then early that morning, a physician she had not met before entered the room and told her she qualified for a very specialized type of treatment that is only applicable in rare circumstances; Bea fit the bill. He was quick to say it would not buy her years, only months, but to her and her family, that was a lifetime.

I ministered to the patient and her family by facilitating a heart-to-heart, end-of-life discussion about the patient's wishes for plan of care.

Secular Spirituality

This group embraces a spiritual philosophy but not a particular religion. They see spirituality as a means for personal growth within a variety of contexts such as self, nature, or others, even death or near-death (Secular Spirituality, 2019).

Ashley, 22 and single, was from a religious family though not particularly spiritual herself, at least not until the night she was raped by a cab driver, thrown out of the car at high speed, then promptly and purposely run over by her assailant and left for dead. A little later at 4:00 a.m., she was nearly hit again as she lay helpless on the dark road, this time by a passing truck, but he braked in time and called 911.

On life support in the ICU, it was touch and go. Her parents were consumed with grief, fear, and anger. She had been run over from the neck down, and survival was questionable.

Over time and with numerous operations, Ashley did survive. She thrived beyond all expectations, with a measure of independence. I spoke to her a few months later when she came in for a follow-up procedure. Her family surrounded her bed and was mesmerized as she spoke through tears of what happened to her and its meaning for her. As a result of her brush with death, she now had a new spiritual life. She believed this was a gift from God to bring her bickering family together. They put petty complaints aside and through the miracle of her survival found forgiveness in their hearts for one another.

Ashley continues to seek her purpose in life. The newfound peace in her family is only the beginning. She is telling her story to others, urging them to embrace the things in life that really matter – to put materialism aside and love the things that are freely given by God.

I ministered to Ashley by facilitating conversation about what that night meant to her and how she is growing from it, finding new meaning in her life, and sharing her story with others.

Seekers

These individuals seek life's meaning and their purpose in it. They are looking for paths that can guide them to truth. Their inspirations and feelings of awe can come from within or from something outside themselves but often relate to a gift (received existentially or externally) that has been given to them to share (Ammerman, 2013).

Jake was raised Catholic but did not consider himself spiritual in the traditional sense. He vacillated between anger at God who let innocent people suffer and thus doubted his existence at all, yet he wanted to believe because he was afraid of what would happen to his soul if he died as a nonbeliever.

He longed for something awe inspiring and peaceful. He saw it in the twinkle of the stars, the majesty of the mountains, and the power of the ocean. He saw it in the little things people did as they went about their lives and the love with which they did it – hairdressers, veterinarians, valet parkers, dog walkers. He saw spirituality in the animals – wild rabbits, puppies, even insects he would capture and take outside to their freedom if found in the house. However, he felt weak and unworthy. He believed that if a power so great did exist, it could not possibly love him.

Jake had been fighting cancer for 18 years, chronic pneumonia for 3, and a host of other complications. He could not eat, talk, smell, walk, or breathe (without oxygen). He had a feeding tube, a trach, and crippled feet. He was in constant pain and fear but fought the notion of hospice and especially do not resuscitate instructions with all his might. Finally, hospice was inevitable when it became obvious the cancer would win the war and there was nothing else the doctors could do. His wife told him if he wanted to live, to make a plan with God and she would support whatever he and God decided.

In hospice, Jake finally opened up about God. He wrote on his pad (his only way of communicating), "I hope there's a heaven. I hope there's a God." I immediately called a priest who came to see Jake. After a long talk about pain and disappointments, near-death experiences, beliefs, and eschatological hopes, Jake opened his arms wide and embraced the priest and the Good Shepherd. At that very moment, he was showered with peace for the first time in years, and that was his best day. His final two weeks were filled with hugs and kisses from his wife, and love and prayer from his family and friends.

He smiled a big smile just before his death, and that was the gift that God gave him to share, assurance that God was taking Jake to a beautiful forever home where there would be peace and no more tears. That smile sustains his wife to this day.

I ministered to the patient by recognizing his Catholic tradition and the values and fears it instilled in him. By calling a priest at end of life, Jake had the chance to make things right with God, whom he had doubted for so long but ultimately embraced in his final days. This brought peace and comfort to his family as well.

Spiritual Nones

The Spiritual Nones consist of various subsets, including atheists, agnostics, and those calling themselves spiritual but with no particular affiliation. Most of this latter category believe in God or a higher power but are not seeking a traditional practice or religious connection. Spiritual Nones is a common selection for patients in the hospital registration process (Schermer, 2018).

George was expected to die that afternoon. George, who was on dialysis, had coded multiple times and was not expected to make it through another session. He was scheduled for dialysis again at 5 p.m. When the machine was turned on, it was anticipated his heart would stop, and the doctors were doubtful they could bring him back. George was fully alert and breathing on his own. I couldn't help but wonder what it would be like to be wide awake and know you were almost certain to die within hours.

George's family had been visiting him throughout the day to say their goodbyes – first his ex-wife, then his preteen children, then his estranged father, and finally me.

When I visited the patient, he told me he had decided to forego his 5 p.m. dialysis session so he could live one more night. Then he leapt to his feelings. His first words were, "I wish I had more time. I was just starting to get it right. I was turning my relationship around with my ex, becoming involved with my kids, and my dad and I were finally starting to talk again. I made a lot of bad decisions in my life that hurt a lot of people, but I am rediscovering God, and my relationship with him is just taking off. I am finally on the right path, but now it is too late."

George went on to say how much one more day would mean to him, that he had just said goodbye to his family for the last time. He had not appreciated what a treasure they were until recently. Now it was all over, wasted, sad. He pleaded, "Just one more day, God, just one more day . . . just one Christmas Day! That is all I ask, Lord. I beg you, please."

At that point, I asked the patient if he believed God would do it for him, to give him more time. He looked me in the eyes with a powerful, desperate, yet confident stare and whispered, "Yes. I do believe," and I said, "Then believe!"

That was a Friday night. When I clocked out at the end of my shift, I thought I would never see George again, that he would be dead in the morning.

When I arrived at work on Monday night, I checked the deceased list, expecting to see George's name. But he wasn't there. I checked all the ICUs, and he wasn't there either, nor was he on the discharge list. I finally found him in the cardiac stepdown unit. I did not know what to expect when I entered his room, but what I saw surprised and delighted me. He was sitting up, eating a plate of chicken pasta, and grinning ear to ear. I checked with his nurse, who said he "did great" in dialysis, as well as anyone there.

I had the opportunity to visit George several times over the next couple of weeks until his discharge to rehab. On our last visit, he told me he speaks to God all the time, that he found the path to truth he was looking for. He said he used to pray only when he was in trouble but never when things were good. Now, he says, he prays every day and always will in good times and in bad since he has rediscovered God and learned that he is real.

I ministered to George by allowing him to believe in a miracle. At that point, it was all he had. He replaced his desolation with hope and unquestionable belief in a God that can do anything. Even had he not made it, his last hours would have been spent with a burning love for God in his heart rather than regret and despair. (Please note, I would not have taken this tactic with the family. Creating false hope among loved ones in a dire situation is cruel.)

Conclusion

The article *Cry Heart But Never Break: A Remarkable Illustrated Meditation on Loss and Life* (Popova, 2016) reviews the celebrated children's book on death and dying by Dutch author Glenn Ringtved (2001). In his book Ringtved presents the Grim Reaper, "Death," as a kindly soul who goes about his mission with a heavy but wise heart. On one particular night, he comes for the grandmother of four little children who live with her in a "small snug house" and who love her dearly. They try to keep Death from his mission by plying him with coffee all night, hoping he will leave without her.

With compassion and dignity, Death helps them see that dying is natural and necessary for new life. "What would life be worth if there were no death?" he asks them. "Who would enjoy the sun if it never rained?"

After their grandmother's soul has flown away, the children surround her bed. They feel a "great moment of sadness, enveloped in warm peacefulness." In the midst of the gentle breeze blowing through the curtains, Death says quietly to the children, "Cry, heart, but never break. Let your tears of grief and sadness help begin new life."

Dying with dignity in the presence of loved ones, free from pain, and at peace with one's beliefs is a good death. With time for peace, reflectiveness, warm words, caresses, even silence can speak volumes as one prepares to transcend or simply cease to be. The act of dying is impartial to philosophies, beliefs, rituals, symbols, science, purpose, and paths. The only truth we can be sure of is that we all go through it. Will yours be a good death?

Discussion Questions

1. Does it matter if a patient is not religious or spiritual or has some similar doctrine by which he or she lives?
2. At the end of life, despite an individual's specific religion, how can chaplains provide a spiritual connection to those individuals who have no religious affiliation?

References

Ammerman, N. T. (2013). Spiritual but not religious? Beyond binary choices in the study of religion. *Journal for the Scientific Study of Religion* 52(2), 259, 269, 270, 274. doi:10.1111/jssr.12024.

Lartey, E. (2006). *Pastoral Theology in an Intercultural World*. Cleveland, OH: Pilgrim Press.

Popova, M. (2016). *Cry, Heart, But Never Break: A Remarkable Illustrated Meditation on Loss and Life*. www.brainpickings.org/2016/03/08/cry-heart-but-never-break/.

Religious Disaffiliation. s.v. Wikipedia. https://en.wikipedia.org/wiki/Religious_disaffiliation, Accessed July 2019.

Ringtved, G. (2001). *Cry, Heart, but Never Break*. Brooklyn, NY: Enchanted Lion Books.

Schermer, M. (2018, April). Silent no more. *Scientific American* 318(4), 77.

Secular Spirituality. s.v. Wikipedia. https://en.wikipedia.org/wiki/Secular_spirituality, Accessed August 2019.

Part 2

Palliative Care and Practice

Chapter 8

Pain, Suffering, and Palliative Sedation

Carlo Casalone

Given modern technological advances and our lengthening life spans, it is almost inevitable that most of us will experience pain towards the end of our lives. But pain – whether of the body, the mind, or the soul – is hard to define, hard to describe. No two people (perhaps not even the same person in different circumstances) experience pain the same way. Pain reminds us we are human and, in so doing, allows us to acknowledge our humanity, permits us to reach beyond ourselves.

It is difficult to develop a discourse about pain, because it concerns an appalling and scandalous experience that does not allow itself to be enclosed in a unitary and orderly boundary. Yet the attempt to speak of this existential issue is fundamental: only the labor of naming and sharing the many resonances that it evokes, however contradictory and shocking it may be, makes it possible to inscribe it, albeit in a way that is never definitive and complete, in a context of meaning. Only by following this itinerary is it made more sustainable, or at least its destructive power is reduced. It is not a solitary enterprise but requires a shared and community investment. Throughout history, cultures have always ventured into this work to which we are urged, even in our highly technological context (Natoli, 1989).

From Natural Sciences to the Question of Meaning

Neither can the function of pain be clearly defined at the level of natural sciences. In fact, it is understood as a signal informing about something that happens in the organism and threatens its integrity. The first to speak in these terms in a scientific frame seems to have been René Descartes, in his treatise *De homine* (published posthumously in the second half of the 17th century): pain is described here as an alarm bell that warns the soul of an imminent danger. Several illustrations of his text show the afferent path of pain. A famous sketch represents a boy with a foot near flames and the ways of transmission of pain that run through the limb and spinal cord to reach the brain. Here we find a first draft of a reflex arc, a sort of feedback that urges the boy to retract his foot (Descartes, 1648, 91; Canguilhem, 1977, 66).

After more than three centuries, Descartes's theory still enjoys great popularity and interprets pain as a sign of damage to which the body is exposed and from which it is necessary to defend itself. Various pathological conditions confirm this approach. Congenital analgesia (an insensitivity to pain) is an emblematic example. Those who are affected by this disease, fortunately very rare, die quite young, since it is impossible for them to make use of this precious warning. However, it is difficult to find a satisfactory definition of pain, since other phenomena do not correspond to this description, and indeed contradict it.[1] First of all, it is not uncommon for pain to come late; not a few diseases, even serious ones, develop without warning. When pain occurs late, the deterioration of the organism can be very advanced and sometimes irreversible: there is damage without pain. On the other hand, in many circumstances, the pain does not allow the body to activate any defense reaction but only makes an impaired situation even more painful. Pain then becomes a disease in itself, particularly when protracted in a chronic form: it "further weakens the subject and makes it more ill than it would be without it," as René Leriche (1937) says in his classic work on surgical pain (quoted in Le Breton, 2010, 11).

Pain therefore shows an enigmatic face, because its function cannot be completely decrypted. Furthermore, the question also arises on the neurophysiological level, since scholars have long debated its genesis: whether pain originates from peripheral nociceptors (i.e., structures specifically dedicated to the detection of pain) or whether its perception is rather determined by the level of intensity with which the nerve endings of the eventually injured tissues are activated or by the type of neuronal (dedicated) pathways that convey the transmission, also subjected to modulation by higher centers. Therefore, pain does not have a univocal role, since it can also be devoid of any purpose and its functioning is not adequately known (Cassel, 2014, 2283). Perhaps it would be more appropriate to speak of "pains," in a plural form, which surface under the appearance of multiple shapes, thus avoiding generalizing that keeps at a distance the concrete and singular situations of those who experience it (Trentin, 2004, 344). In any case, the impossibility of identifying a clear and satisfactory explanation pushes us to situate our question within a further horizon and to develop the discourse on another level.

From the Empirical Approach to the Lived Experience

Turning now to the "firsthand" experience of pain, it is difficult to clearly define limits with respect to how it is experienced; it is very difficult to discriminate if it comes from the *body* or from the *soul* (Le Breton, 2010, 13–29).

The subjective resonances evoked by pain are sometimes defined as suffering, which would therefore indicate its inner repercussion on a psychological and existential level. In palliative care, the expression coined by Cicely Saunders of "total pain" (Turriziani & Zaninetta, 2018, 329) is also employed to indicate the involvement of the whole of the person, inextricably weaving pain, anxiety, and anguish. On the philosophical level, others make a distinction between *damage* (although we have seen that pain is not always related to organic damage) and *meaning* (Natoli, 2015, 57–58). Lived pain or experience of suffering arises between harm (physical dimension) and meaning (existential dimension). The damage is, in fact, differently interpreted in different belief systems and in individual cultures. Human communities have provided linguistic, symbolic, and ritual resources to cope with this experience, which radically questions the flourishing of life in its spontaneous evidence. In fact, each of us originally belongs to a culture within which we find the references to orient ourselves in existence. Pain interrupts this usual perception of the experienced world, introducing a contradiction and raising questions: "Why me?" "What did I do to deserve this suffering?" "Why did I receive a life that is now so severely impaired or even stolen from me?" Depending on its intensity and gravity, it can go so far as to disrupt one's overall sense of the world.

Although the damage is universally recognizable and empirically measurable, the meaning is rather particular, because it depends on the person and the culture he or she belongs to. Materially ascertainable, different experiences of suffering can correspond to the same damage, based also on the modulation induced by the context. In the realization of a project and in the motivated trust in a promise of the meaning of life, different forms of lack and suffering find meaning and are handled with courage. The volunteers who rush to serve on the occasion of a natural catastrophe endure with less effort discomforts and pains, even physical ones, as they support them better, "suffer" them less. This applies to every struggle faced in the name of a cause or of a loved one.

These subjective differences are to be attributed also to the fact that everyone is immersed in a scenario of meaning from which he or she is preceded, starting from birth. In pain we look for words to give meaning to what seems absurd, and the culture in which each one finds him/herself provides expressions and symbols to interpret the contradiction of pain, nevertheless knowing that it is never possible to resolve its unspeakable depth. The two most ancient and relevant scenarios in the Mediterranean basin are the Greek-Roman and Jewish-Christian traditions. In the first, pain is connatural to life, and therefore it can only be stemmed and endured through science and virtue; in the second, it is interpreted not only as a natural fact but also as a historical event related to human freedom and therefore can be defeated and redeemed (Rizzi, 1995, 83–87). The difficulty then consists in succeeding, through pain, in giving meaning to life even when injured, recognizing solidarity in common exposure to the imponderable. The experience of pain has therefore an objective side, where damage and illness are positioned, and a personal and cultural side, which refers to the meaning in which pain can be elaborated, without hiding the radical reaction of rejection and rebellion that it arouses.

The Techno-Scientific Scenario of Today's Medicine

Techno-science introduces profound changes in the scenario in which pain is experienced. It generates other references of meaning, other expectations on the part of patients and healthcare workers, and provides hitherto unknown tools for dealing with it. This role of medical activity is nothing new; already in the work of Hippocrates it is argued that the doctor and the patient must work together in the search for causes, meaning, and treatment of pain (Rey, 2011, 30). But today's change consists of the quality and power of the tools that techno-science makes available. Medicine has experienced a phase of expansion and increasing efficacy: life in all phases is subjected to its intervention and to its control. It has also modified, with sophisticated conceptual and operational tools, a reduction of the body to organism, in a mechanistic view. Cognitive objectivation and intervention of technique have favored the marginalization of the word and the failure to listen to the symptom as a signal that refers to deeper levels of existence.

Medical intervention, with its complexity, while seeking health, also appears as a constraint that breaks into the life of the sick person and further aggravates the pain, being in turn a cause of suffering (Marin, 2011). We can indicate at least three levels in which such an intrusion occurs. The first impact takes place at the level of the organizational environment in which care is given. The hospital is a foreign space in which time is articulated on the schedules of diagnostic and therapeutic processes, forcing patients to change their usual habits and rhythms. Second, the treatment of the body is subjected to technical procedures, laboratory investigations, and interventions that disrupt the border of the skin lining and the internal volumes of the organism, ordinarily reserved and kept in intimacy. Finally, the psychic dimension is affected, since decisions need to be made, constraints that reduce the margins of autonomy, confronted with a difficult and objectifying language, such as can be seen in expressions such as "How is your leg?" or "How is your breath doing?" or "We'll do an abdomen echograph." Even pain therapy continually risks losing sight of the relationship with the painful person. The expression itself may indicate a dangerous reductionism. Of course, practical needs require the use of synthetic and functional expressions. Yet, even from an etymological point of view, "pain therapy" is quite problematic. The Greek verb *therapeuein* has a much greater amplitude than that entailed in this formulation. In fact, three levels can be indicated: the original meaning indicates the action of giving someone *service and honor*; therefore, it contains a similar connotation as *to render honor and respect*, also in the religious sense of worship, referring to the gods. From this first meaning springs the second, which indicates *taking care*. Finally, the third refers to *medicating successfully* and then *healing*. So speaking about *pain therapy* is misleading for two reasons: first of all because it neglects the original meaning we have described, focusing on the secondary significances, and second, because pain does not exist as an abstract entity, but only painful people exist, with their specific singularity in perceiving the damage that afflicts the organism. In a climate of struggle against the disease, the patient as a subject is roughly pushed to the margins. The perspective is therefore to fight the limit represented by the disease, as it also anticipates the radical limit of death – a very fruitful perspective that allows us to overcome formerly lethal pathologies but which risks obscuring the constitutive finiteness and vulnerability that are characteristic to the human condition.

Medical Intervention: Limits and Relationships

In the end, medicine today also shows signs of being willing to recognize and accept limitations. This happens above all in the growing awareness that the ability to treat acute diseases often leads to the production of chronic pathological situations. The gap between diagnostic and therapeutic capacities is widening, so that increasing the expectation of life prolongs the time of cohabitation with diseases. Think of the human immunodeficiency virus (HIV) infection: in the 1980s, it left a few years of life to those who were affected, while today, the infection can be controlled until death, which happens from other causes. Furthermore, by resorting more and more to prostheses and bionic materials that supplant or support physiological activities that our organs are no longer able to perform, we face long periods of treatment for multiple pathologies. A second aspect of awareness is constituted by pain therapy and palliative care, two related practices, even if they do not coincide. They attest to the conviction that even though healing is not always possible, it is still possible to take care of the person.

Therefore, it is a matter of assuming a certain coefficient of impotence, even symbolic, which is particularly difficult in the age of technical efficiency, centered on control and performance – an attitude that requires a laborious rereading of the experience of the caregivers, called to familiarize themselves with limits and mortality (Desmet, 2004). Palliative medicine, and the culture behind it, says that in today's (Western) world, it is possible to talk about relationships, communication, dialogue, and fears evoked by pain and illness, working effectively to maintain and re-establish bonds where the pain tears them apart and interrupts them (Orsi, 2018, 89–96; Pontifical Academy for Life, 2019). If pain separates, life is a bond, and bonds help us to live. They stand up to suffering because not all of them have yet broken, and the still-labile threads make it possible to re-weave life. There is a need not to feel alone, to establish communication through the word. Of course, delicacy is needed: it is important to carefully calibrate the dialogue on the patient's questions without being intrusive. The ability to be connected nurtures an instinctive competence to find the right moment to start an interview; what is at stake is not a technique but an attitude of empathy and compassion. In this climate of relationship, even the person who suffers can find glimpses in order not to remain in the narrow world in which the pain tends to enclose her. Acknowledging the presence and humanity of the other, she finds reasons to live and to freely give her life in whatever time remains, and in giving, she can live. It is therefore a question of addressing to those who suffer words and tones that communicate that they are important, that their dignity is not crushed by the disease. This not only motivates them but empowers them to live: If you die, I will die. Living becomes a responsibility for those who suffer. Identifying the threads that can reassemble a plot of proximity is the way to belong to each other and to face the difficult choices that can occur in the imminence of death.

It is important that medical interventions to treat pain not obscure this context. The prescription of analgesics does not exclude the continuous search for ways to meet all the dimensions of life of the sick person, which also affects the experience of pain. Palliative care has fostered a holistic approach to all the needs of the patient. For this reason, a careful discernment is necessary in order to proceed with sedation, especially when prolonged and deep, in the terminal phase (Bruera, 2012; Cherny, 2009; Rodrigues, 2018). It is a particularly demanding choice for the sick, for family members, and for the caregivers. That's why it must be included in a communicative and decision-making process that involves everyone according to the role she or he plays. In fact, in this case, it will suppress "the relational and communicative dimension that we saw as crucial in accompanying palliative care. . . . Sedation is therefore always at least partially unsatisfactory, and it must be considered as an extreme remedy, to be adopted only after having carefully examined and clarified all relevant factors" (Francis, 2018).

The Technical "Doing" and the Elaboration of Meaning

The tools of medicine can and must be introduced from a perspective that is not reduced to technical "doing." They can be deliberately assumed in a responsible action as mediations within a language that, in our world, as has always happened in the past and continues to occur in every culture, contributes to the processing of suffering. History attests that human beings, faced with the events and contradictions that question life, have been continuously searching for meaning and have found new resources to reaffirm it. This happened not only due to the abilities of single individuals but also because living consists of belonging to a horizon of meaning that is already present and precedes us as we enter the world. Language is the most explicit expression of this precedent context: We find it already in place, and we are inserted into it. When we are born, we also learn about the symbolic mediations that the community in which we find ourselves uses in its confrontation with suffering. Since humanity has gone through the centuries and still lasts over time, it means that it was able to find, if not answers to suffering, at least possibilities of resistance and good reasons to continue living without closing itself to transformation.

Thus, the task of integrating the undeniable and positive progress that medicine has made without neglecting the quality of relationships is outlined, without denying the limit but rather including it and thus recognizing impotence even in the new cultural situation we are living in. Certainly, mitigating violent pain, preventing it from obscuring any other experience so that any other question is prevented, is a service that science and technology can commendably render. The conditions in which we live make it increasingly likely that everyone will witness the spectacle of her or his own progressive decline. It is not only a benefit but also a more provoking situation: long periods of illness, being aware of the ineluctable outcome. The inseparable link between physical pain and existential suffering is emphasized by this situation. Today, too, as in every culture, we are called to recognize how the power of life and its meaning are stronger than suffering, as all cultures have committed themselves to cope with wounds of existence and of coexistence. The answers will be historically shaped and therefore may be incomplete or even not entirely correct, as was the case of giving to pain in itself a redeeming function in the Christian tradition. But on the other side, this same tradition provided enormous contributions about this topic, as it continues to do, drawing on the ever-new resources of faith experience. Challenged by the laceration of suffering, clinical activity is urged to insert itself in the context of right relationships, allowing everyone to experience a reciprocity that offers good reasons to live.

Discussion Questions

1. Give an example of personal factors that have effects on end-of-life decision-making.
2. How can technical activity be fruitfully integrated into the elaboration of the meaning of suffering?

Note

1. The definition of pain from the International Association for the Study of Pain (IASP) sounds like this: "An unpleasant sensory and emotional experience associated with actual or potential tissue damage, or described in terms of such damage" (www.iasp-pain.org/Education/Content.aspx?ItemNumber=1698, Accessed September 22, 2019). Sometimes we talk about pain as "an awareness of a nociceptive message," but even the cores of these definitions, including that of Descartes, are not entirely satisfactory.

References

Bruera, E. (2012, April). Sedation when and how? *Journal of Clinical Oncology* 30(12), 1258–1259.

Canguilhem, G. (1977). *La Formation du concept de réflexe aux xviiie et xviii e siècles*. Paris: Vrin.

Cassel, E. J. (2014). *Pain and suffering*. In B. Jennings (Ed.), *Encyclopedia of Bioethics*, 4th ed., Vol. 5, 2283–2291. New York: Cengage Learning, Macmillan.

Cherny, N., et al. (2009). European Association for Palliative Care (EAPC) recommended framework for the use of sedation in palliative care. *Palliative Medicine* 23, 581–593.

Descartes, R. (1648). *Traité de l'homme*. Cited in Rey, R. (2011). *Histoire de la douleur*. Paris: La Découverte.

Desmet, M. (2004). La dynamique de l'expérience médicale. Une relecture biblique. In O. Artus et al. (Eds.), *Bible et médecine. Le corps et l'esprit*, 101–139. Brussels: Presses Universitaires de Namur – Lessius.

Francis, Pope. (2018, February 28). Letter on the Occasion of the Palliative Care Conference. Organized by the Pontifical Academy for Life, Rome.

Le Breton, D. (2010). *Expériences de la douleur. Entre destruction et renaissance*. Paris: Métailié.

Leriche, R. (1937). *Chirurgie de la douleur*. Paris: Masson.

Marin, C. (2011). Violence de la maladie, violence dans le soin. In P. Verspieren & M. S. Richard (Eds.), *Violence dans la maladie, violence dans le soin*, 15–31. Paris: Mediasèvres.

Natoli, S. (1989). *L'esperienza del dolore. Le forme del patire nella cultura occidentale*. Milan: Feltrinelli.

Natoli, S. (2015). Giobbe, lo scandalo del dolore. In C. M. Martini (Ed.), *Le cattedre dei non credenti*, 57–74. Milan: Bompiani.

Orsi, L. (2018). *Il dolore. Parole per capire, ascoltare, capirsi*. Milano: In dialogo.

Pontifical Academy for Life. (2019). *White Book for Global Palliative Care Advocacy*. Rome: PAV.

Rey, R. (2011). *Histoire de la douleur*. Paris: La Découverte.

Rizzi, A. (1995). *Il Sacro e il Senso. Lineamenti di filosofia della religione*. Leumann, TO: Elle Di Ci.

Rodrigues, P., et al. (2018). Palliative sedation for existential suffering: A systematic review of argument-based ethics literature. *Journal of Pain and Symptom Management* 55, 1577–1590.

Trentin, G. (2004). Dolore. In S. Leone & S. Privitera (Eds.), *Nuovo Dizionario di Bioetica*, 344–348. Rome: Città Nuova.

Turriziani, A., & Zaninetta, G. (2018). *Il mondo delle cure palliative*. Bologna: Esculapio.

Chapter 9

Compassionate Presence

The Accompaniment of Patients and Families in the Midst of Their Suffering

Christina M. Puchalski

In many parts of the world, patients today are served by health systems geared toward their technical care, where little regard is given to other aspects of their treatment. This problem is compounded by societal concerns about what is appropriate. Although board-certified chaplains as well as spiritual care professionals are available, such spiritual care is often left to physicians and healthcare professionals who may lack the time or training to deal with these "extras." Rooted in philosophy and theology, compassionate presence allows patients and families to deal with the trials facing them in a way that provides spiritual understanding and acceptance.

As a medical student on the wards each morning, I visited my patients to prepare to present their updated condition during formal morning rounds. One morning, I could not find one of my very ill patients, whom I will call Alice. The nurse told me that Alice had been moved down the hall away from the "busy nursing station" so that she could have more "peace and quiet" because there was "nothing more we could do for her." When I entered her new room, I saw three empty beds and, in the corner, my patient lying on the fourth bed. She was curled up in a semi-fetal position, quietly sobbing. Her thin, frail face was partially buried in a starkly white hospital pillow. I pulled a chair up to her bed, conscious of the loud scratchy noise the chair made in this hollow large room. I asked Alice how she was doing. No answer, just quiet sobs. I reached out and held her hand. After some time in silence, she said she felt so afraid, so lonely, and confused. "Why?" she cried out. "Why? I thought I was getting better." Her despair was palpable. I felt helpless at first, but as I held her hand and listened, the intensity of her despair seemed to lessen a bit. At the end of our time together, she thanked me for listening to her. Her tears seemed to abate. She was able to answer a few medical questions I asked. It was clear to me that the most important concern was the existential questions of "Why me?" and "Why now?"

I have often reflected on what would have happened to her and to me if I had plowed through with biomedical questions. What if I had run out, thinking there was "nothing more to do?" In fact, what I learned by sitting with my patient is that there is so much we can and must do for our patients that is not purely biomedical but that can have biomedical consequences. In the case of my patient, she was suffering deeply, and more spiritually than physically. Studies have demonstrated that spiritual or existential distress is associated with increased depression and anxiety, increased physical pain, and worse quality of life (Delgado-Guay et al., 2016; des Ordons et al., 2018). *Guidelines in Palliative Care*, which focuses on the care of seriously and chronically ill patients and those who are dying, requires addressing spiritual issues with patients as a core element of clinical care (Puchalski et al., 2009; Clinical Practice Guidelines, 2018). The World Health Assembly's resolution on palliative care states that it is an "ethical responsibility of health systems, and an ethical duty of health care professionals to alleviate pain and suffering, whether physical, psychosocial or spiritual" (World Health Organization, 2014). Finally, clinical models for integration of interprofessional spiritual care demonstrate how clinicians can assess for and treat spiritual distress and how clinicians can work with spiritual care professionals to fully attend to the spiritual distress of patients (Puchalski, Vitillo, Hull, & Reller, 2014). In these models, an important way to "treat" suffering in patients and their families is by accompanying them on their illness journey and by being fully present to them in all of their suffering – especially the spiritual and existential suffering.

Suffering, in the current medical system, is largely viewed as physical suffering. The current medical model is influenced by the Cartesian dualism model, where in the 19th and 20th centuries, physical pain was relegated to physicians who took care of the body, while spiritual suffering was related to religious leaders, shamans, and other healers. Thus, in that type of model, the focus is on objective laboratory data and physical examination findings, not on patients' stories, beliefs, and values. Medical care is still influenced by the Cartesian dualism model, resulting in making gathering objective data the goal of physicians. In recent years, there has been greater focus on listening to the patients' stories, such as in narrative medicine, and spirituality and health. With the ongoing challenges of time, increased automation with electronic databases, and discussion about artificial intelligence replacing much of a clinician's time with patients, there is increasingly less implementation of what might be considered the softer side of medicine – that is, being present and listening to the whole of the patient, mind, body, and spirit. Eric Cassel wrote of this struggle, noting that "Attempting to understand what suffering is and how physicians might truly be devoted to its relief will require that medicine and its critics overcome the dichotomy between mind and body" (Cassel, 1998). Betty Ferrell and Nessa Coyle, in their book *Suffering and the Goals of Nursing* (2008), note that nurses are continually exposed to suffering, and while they bear witness to the suffering of others, they rarely address their own suffering. Nurses also are exposed to the same pressures of current health systems, and due to time pressures must focus on the physical aspect of care. Ferrell and Coyle's poignant definition of suffering – "Occurring when an individual feels voiceless. This may occur when the person is mute to give words to their experience or when their screams are unheard" – underscores the need for a more holistic approach to attend to the suffering of our patients and their families.

There are other societal occurrences that are working against a purely technically driven health system. The first is the high degree of burnout and moral distress among physicians and nurses, with physician suicide rates being among the highest in all professions. Studies suggest that the reason for this is that physicians and nurses feel conflicted when they cannot do what they love most – being with patients, forming relationships with patients, and providing care for all of the concerns of their patients, not just the physical concerns. The lack of meaning in one's profession can lead to severe spiritual distress and to depression. The second societal concern is patient satisfaction with care. Numerous surveys indicate that patients want to be listened to and that the majority of patients want their spiritual issues addressed (Selman et al., 2018). Third, the increased legalization of assisted suicide is sparking discussion on dignity of life and on what message is given to care for people who are not as functional physical, mentally, or socially as they used to be. I would postulate that the drive behind assisted suicide is stemming from a purely functional physical and mental perspective as to what one considers a valuable member of society. When people are no longer viewed as valuable, that affects their perception of meaning in their life and could lead to severe existential and spiritual distress. Hence, it is not surprising that one of the highest reasons for requests for assisted suicide is existential and spiritual distress. The fourth social occurrence is a huge interest in mindfulness and spirituality. This, I believe, reflects the need for meaning, peace, and connection to the significant or sacred, however people come to understand that for themselves. A key element of mindfulness practice as rooted in contemplative religious and spiritual traditions is being present to oneself and others. These societal occurrences are the opportunity for greater inclusion of compassionate presence in all aspects of life, particularly in the accompaniment of our patients with serious and chronic illness and also at end of life.

The clinical model of interprofessional spiritual care is based on a generalist–specialist model where all clinicians are generalist–spiritual care providers, while board-certified chaplains or spiritual care professionals are the experts in this area. Suffering in this model is viewed both clinically and philosophically. From the clinical perspective, spiritual distress is defined as a diagnosis and includes meaninglessness, hopelessness, despair, conflict with religious beliefs, separation from the transcendent, need for reconciliation, and need for rituals. While this approach is reductionist, it has made inroads in clinical care because it makes philosophical and theological concepts accessible in the clinical setting. Spiritual distress as a clinical definition of suffering can be as "simple" as meaninglessness, despair, or conflict with religious beliefs. But each of these diagnostic words to describe suffering has complex theological, philosophical, and humanistic underpinnings. Generalist–spiritual care professionals need not have theological training to recognize these categories of distress and to be present to the patient as that patient shares their suffering. However, specialist spiritual care professionals do have theological, philosophical, and humanistic training and therefore are able to explore spiritual distress in greater depth with patients. In this way, reductionism is only an opening to profound human interactions and explorations.

The concept of compassionate presence is relatively new within clinical care, unlike the term *compassion*. Gilbert (2010) defined compassion as "suffering with or a deep awareness of the suffering of another coupled with a desire to help the physical mental or emotional of the other." Sinclair et al. (2017) defined it as "a virtuous response that seeks to address suffering and the needs of a person through relational understanding and action." Although much has been written on compassion, little has been written on compassionate presence and its applications clinically. Compassionate presence is a unique subset of compassionate care. It refers to the contemplative aspect of our relationship with patients. While compassionate care can involve empathy, forming connections, helping patients with issues, being respectful, caring, and so forth, compassionate presence calls upon a unique set of skills in which the clinician moves to a more reflective and contemplative space with the patient. Accompaniment, then, is the outgrowth of being present. It is the spiritual work clinicians do. It is spirituality in action at its very depth.

This concept of compassionate presence is not rooted only in philosophy and theology. In clinical care, Munhall (1993) described the concept of unknowing as "being open to the essence of the meaning the patient presents" about the situation and not trying to interpret the meaning of what the patient shares within the clinician's frame of reference, as clinicians might do in more biomedical contexts. Presence in mystical interfaith traditions is described as being present to the divine with neither a cognitive nor an emotional awareness of the divine's presence (*The Collected Works of John of the Cross*, 1979). Thus, compassionate presence involves not just awareness of the presence of the other person but also of the transcendent in the relationship between the clinician and the patient and/or family. This requires an awareness by the clinician of their own sense of transcendence or the divine to be able to recognize that in the clinical encounter with their patients. How was I aware of the divine in my encounter with Alice when I was a student? It originates from my experience as a child in the context of my religious practice as a Catholic. As I was preparing for receiving Communion for the first time as a child, I struggled with the concept of transubstantiation and asked my father, Anthony Puchalski, my most important spiritual teacher, how a piece of bread could be God. He simply said that I was overthinking it and that next time I was in church during the Liturgy of the Eucharist, he invited me to open my heart and be present to the experience and not try to understand it intellectually. When I went to church that week, I experienced a deep sense of God's presence that filled me with awe, wonder, and a love that is hard to describe. I recognized that same presence in the room with my patient. My only response was one of silent reverence for Alice as she shared her pain. We each find a place within our own spiritual experiences that helps us recognize the sacred or divine in others. That is, I believe, essential to move into deep presence with another.

In 2009, George Washington University's Institute for Spirituality and Health (GWish) held a consensus conference on competencies in spirituality and health education using the Accreditation Council for Graduate Medical Education (ACGME) competencies for medical residency education as the framework. These competencies include system-based practices, medical knowledge, practice-based learning, interpersonal and communication skills, and professionalism (Puchalski, Blatt, Kogan, & Butler, 2014). For the practice of compassionate presence, however, the group could not find a specific ACGME competency that completely aligned with compassionate presence; compassionate presence was in part a communication skill, part of patient care, and also part of professional development, as students need to have an awareness of their own spirituality and their vocation to serve in order to be able to accompany patients, especially in the midst of suffering. Thus, the group created its own specific competency on compassionate presence. Key competencies in this category include an awareness of one's vocation to serve, of one's own spirituality, and of the transformative potential of the clinician–patient relationship. This later aspect for me was clearly present with my patient Alice. By being present to another person, we are changed in the encounter at many levels. Alice impacted the way I treat my patients and others and also my call to help teach this practice to my students and health professionals.

Specific communication behaviors for compassionate presence include the practice of deep listening, curious inquiry, perceptive reflections, the use of silence in patient communication, and assessing for spiritual distress. Finally, the overall behavioral competency in which all of the other competency behaviors were framed was practicing medicine as a spiritual practice. This raises awareness of the sacred nature of the relationship between clinicians and their patients. When witnessing moments of deep presence with my patients, many of my students describe those moments as "sense of the holy or divine" and experience a transcendence, deep connection, and sense of profound love. Many spoke of the difficulty to describe what they witnessed and felt: what I often call the experience of mystery.

Two of these concepts – transcendence and mystery – are what makes this practice of compassionate presence challenging to teach and to integrate into clinical care. It lacks the simplicity of reductionism, yet it speaks to the core of the complexity of the human person who is suffering. Cassel (1998) wrote that "Transcendence is probably the most powerful way in which one is restored to wholeness after an injury to personhood. When experienced, transcendence locates the person in a far larger landscape. The sufferer is not isolated by pain but is brought closer to a transpersonal source of meaning and to the human community that shares those meanings. Such an experience need not involve religion in any formal sense; however, in its transpersonal dimension, it is deeply spiritual." It speaks to how we can help "treat" suffering, particularly spiritual distress. As we accompany people on their illness journeys, we come upon significant touch points – times when the suffering is intense, as it was for my patient previously. During these times, it is critical that we move away from our biomedical focus to a reflective, contemplative one and practice compassionate presence. Two models for teaching and practicing compassionate presence are the GRACE model of Roshi Joan Halifax (2018) and a model I have developed based on Lectio Divina, a contemplative Christian meditation that dates back to the early mothers and fathers of the church (Puchalski, 2020). In both of these models, there is a preparatory stage, where the clinician focuses their attention on the present moment with the patient, followed by awareness of their intent to serve the other, then attuning to the patient, and transitioning to silence to give space to the patient to share – without any attempt to fix, interpret, or judge and by using contemplative listening skills and reflective inquiry as appropriate. The clinician uses their awareness/intuition to transition back to the other aspect of the clinical care.

Compassionate presence addresses the concerns of the four societal movements discussed earlier. Burnout of clinicians can be mitigated by integrating the spiritual focus even more fully in medical education, helping clinicians learn how to practice loving presence and accompaniment within busy clinical settings. Students and clinicians alike experience less burnout and a greater sense of meaning when they are able to connect deeply with their patients. Deep listening, which is a part of compassionate presence, results in patients feeling heard; doing a spiritual assessment meets the need of many patients to have their spiritual concerns addressed in the clinical setting and also helps the clinician identify spiritual distress. One of the major reasons for aid-in-dying requests is spiritual and existential distress, which often is labeled as not being able to be treated (Peled, Bickel, & Puchalski, 2017). Yet compassionate presence and authentic accompaniment help the patient come to an understanding of their own suffering and often a resolution of that suffering. Finally, the increased interest in mindfulness and spirituality can help promote greater understanding and practice of compassionate presence in all settings.

Palliative care is a model of clinical care that is based on the whole-person model of care, or what Cicely Saunders, the founder of hospice and palliative care, called attending to the "total pain" of the patient – psychosocial and spiritual as well as physical (Clark, 1999). It is critically important that as palliative care continues to develop globally, spiritual care be not only part of palliative care but the foundation of palliative care. Spiritual care is premised on the belief that all people – regardless of physical, intellectual, emotional, social, and spiritual health status – have an inherent value and meaning that should be honored and respected through all of life and through natural dying.

But as with all of healthcare today, palliative care is also challenged with lack of resources, human and financial. In the majority of the world, there are no trained spiritual healthcare professionals, such as board-certified chaplains. Clinicians are stretched to their limits with large patient volumes, and the majority of clinicians are not yet trained in attending to the spiritual dimensions of their patients' lives. Studies have shown that the main reason for not attending to the spiritual issues of patients is lack of training in spiritual care (Balboni et al., 2017).

To help bridge the gap of need for spiritual care training in palliative care, George Washington University's Institute for Spirituality and Health developed several programs. The first program, Interprofessional Spiritual Care Education Curriculum (ISPEC) for healthcare professionals, is a new multi-year, outcomes-based education initiative to improve spiritual care for patients with serious and chronic illness. ISPEC trains interdisciplinary teams of clinicians, physicians, nurses, social workers, psychologists, physical and occupational therapists, and spiritual care providers to recognize, address, and attend to the spiritual needs and suffering of patients with chronic and serious illness and that of their families. Critical to achieving these outcomes is a culture change where dignity, respect, and compassion form the foundation of care. Based on the generalist–specialist model of care and the National Coalition for Hospice and Palliative Care (NCP) guidelines (John of the Cross, 1979), all team members are responsible for addressing patient suffering and providing support to patients and families.

The Interprofessional Spiritual Care Education Curriculum includes three components:

- Online training program: This training focuses on knowledge building using case-based learning, virtual presentations, videos, and reading materials. One of the online modules is on compassionate presence.
- Train-the-trainer program: A two-day program focusing on leadership skills, effecting institutional culture change, goal development, integration of spiritual care into clinical practice and education, and assessment and care planning. Participants receive one year of mentoring post-course. Formal program evaluation occurs at 6 and 12 months post-course.
- ISPEC for institutions: The program offers training within a single institution to equip clinicians and chaplains with leadership skills to advance uniform implementation of spiritual care.

ISPEC has been offered in the United States with participants from the United States and 15 other countries. It has also been offered in Australia and Rwanda at the respective annual palliative care meetings and in Chile (Puchalski et al., 2019).

The second program is called GWish Reflection Rounds (G-RR), which was piloted in 18 medical schools (Puchalski et al., 2014). This program was developed as a way to teach the competency behaviors of compassionate presence as described previously. Based on the evaluation of these 18 programs, students who complete G-RR have an increased awareness of their own spirituality, of the importance of the physician–patient relationship, and of their call to serve patients. Students also note that they experience compassionate listening in the small groups, which in turn helps them practice that type of listening with their patients. G-RR is a mentored small-group program for medical students that is integrated into the mainstream clinical rounding system. The G-RR process is unique, as it is designed to nurture students' inner and spiritual professional growth through a contemplative reflection process based on group spiritual direction. It is facilitated by teams of specially trained physicians, chaplains, and counseling professionals such as social workers. Students structure narratives around a modified verbatim format derived from chaplain training. The main focus is on spiritual formation as part of professional formation. Accompanying patients in the midst of their suffering requires clinicians to have an awareness of their own sense of the sacred, an ability to listen deeply, and the inner strength not to take on the suffering of the other. As Pope Francis said in his address to the bishops in Brazil in 2013,

> It is important to devise and ensure a suitable formation, one that will provide persons able to step into the night without being overcome by the darkness and losing their bearings; able to listen to people's dreams without being seduced and to share their disappointments without losing hope and becoming bitter; able to sympathize with the brokenness of others without losing their own strength and identity.
>
> (Pope Francis, Address to Brazilian bishops, July 27, 2013)

This program, integrated throughout clinical training, aims to provide that type of formation for clinicians. It is important for the formation of palliative care practitioners to include this inner formation as a required part of teaching the ministry of accompaniment, the ministry of presence.

Finally, as evident from the chaplain–clinician partnerships of the previous two programs, spiritual care professionals are critically important to the provision of spiritual care. Thus, these programs have resulted in a greater demand for spiritual care professionals. Our partners, including the Association for Clinical Pastoral Education (ACPE), several chaplaincy organizations in the United States, and the European Research Institute for Chaplains in Healthcare (ERICH) in Europe, are working on culturally appropriate models of clinical pastoral education to help train and develop spiritual care professionals globally to increase access to specialist spiritual care professionals. This will greatly impact the care patients receive in several ways, including having spiritual care professionals partnering with clinicians for training programs such as ISPEC and providing leadership training in spiritual care in palliative care with their clinician colleagues. As reflective professional development programs that include spirituality as part of those programs develop in other countries, these spiritual care professionals will be the specialized mentors for the groups such as G-RR.

Mother Teresa noted that while "we can cure physical disease with medicine, the only cure for loneliness, despair, and hopelessness is love. There are many in the world who are dying for a piece of bread but there are many more dying for a little love." Accompaniment is the loving practice of compassionate presence. It is the essential basis of spiritual care and thus of palliative care. By developing spiritually centered palliative care, where all clinicians and caregivers practice from their deep sense of vocation to serve others, honor the dignity of those they serve, and find the sacred in caring for their patients, people with serious illness and their families will be able to find healing, hope, and a sense of peace.

Dedicated to my father, Anthony Puchalski, an incredibly devoted father, a wise teacher, and a holy and fully present man – my inspiration for creating healthcare systems that promote healing and wholeness through the full integration of spiritual care.

References

Balboni, T. A., Fitchett, G., Handzo, G. F., et al. (2017). State of the science of spirituality and palliative care research. Part II: Screening, assessment, and interventions. *Journal of Pain and Symptom Management* 54, 441–453.

Cassel, E. (1998). The nature of suffering and the goals of medicine. *Loss, Grief, and Care* 8(1–2), 129–142.

Clark, D. (1999) "Total pain," disciplinary power and the body in the work of Cicely Saunders, 1958–1967. *Social Science and Medicine* 49, 727–736.

Clinical Practice Guidelines for Quality Palliative Care. (2018). *Domain 5: Spiritual, Religious, and Existential Aspects of Care.* Alexandria, VA: National Coalition for Hospice and Palliative Care.

Delgado-Guay, M. O., Chisholm, G., Williams, J., et al. (2016). Frequency, intensity, and correlates of spiritual pain in advanced cancer patients assessed in a supportive/palliative care clinic. *Palliative and Supportive Care* 14, 341–348.

des Ordons, A., Sinuff, T., Stelfox, H., et al. (2018). Spiritual distress within inpatient settings – A scoping review of patient and family experiences. *Journal of Pain and Symptom Management* 156, 122–145.

Ferrell, B. R., & Coyle, N. (2008). The nature of suffering and the goals of nursing. *Oncology Nursing Forum* 35(2), 241–247.

Gilbert, P. (2010). *The Compassionate Mind: A New Approach to Life's Challenges.* Oakland, CA: New Harbinger.

Halifax, J. (2018). *Standing on the Edge: Finding Freedom Where Fear and Courage Meet.* New York: Flatiron Books.

Kavanagh, K., & Rodriguez, O. (1979). *The Collected Works of St. John of the Cross.* Washington, DC: Institute of Carmelite Studies. Book One, Chapter 12.

Munhall, P. L. (1993). "Unknowing": Toward another pattern of knowing in nursing. *Nursing Outlook* 41, 125–128.

Peled, H., Bickel, K., & Puchalski, C. (2017). Enhancing informed consent for physician aid in dying: Potential role of handout on possible benefits of palliative care. *Journal of Oncology Practice*. http://dx.doi.org/10.1200/JOP.2017.021105.

Pope Francis. (2013, July 27). *Address to Brazilian bishops*. http://w2.vatican.va/content/francesco/en/speeches/2013/july/documents/papa-francesco_20130727_gmg-episcopato-brasile.html.

Puchalski, C. (2020). Lectio Divina model of compassionate presence. JPSM Section on Humanities, Art, Language and Spirituality, manuscript in preparation.

Puchalski, C. M., Blatt, B., Kogan, M., & Butler, A. (2014). Spirituality and health: The development of a field. *Academic Medicine* 89(1), 10–16.

Puchalski, C. M., Ferrell, B., Virani, R., et al. (2009). Improving the quality of spiritual care as a dimension of palliative care: The report of the consensus conference. *Journal of Palliative Medicine* 12, 885–904.

Puchalski, C. M., Jafari, N., Buller, H., et. al. (2019). Interprofessional spiritual care education curriculum. *Journal of Palliative Medicine*. doi:10.1089/jpm.2019.0375.

Puchalski, C. M., Vitillo, R., Hull, S. K., & Reller, N. (2014). Improving the spiritual dimension of whole person care: Reaching national and international consensus. *Journal of Palliative Medicine* 17, 642–656.

Selman, L. E., Brighton, L. J., Sinclair, S., et al. (2018). Patients' and caregivers' needs, experiences, preferences and research priorities in spiritual care: A focus group study across nine countries. *Palliative Medicine* 32, 216–230.

Sinclair, S. et al. (2017). Can self-compassion promote healthcare provider well-being and compassionate care to others? Results of a systematic review applied psychology. *Health and Well-Being* 9(2), 168–206.

World Health Organization. (2014). *Strengthening of Palliative Care as a Component of Comprehensive Care Throughout the Life Course: Resolution WHA67.19*. Geneva: World Health Organization.

Chapter 10

Evidence-Based Communication in the Palliative Conversation

Ways of Restoring Dignity by Simple Actions

Kimberson Tanco and Eduardo Bruera

Accurate and responsible communication is key, especially when deliver-ing information regarding end-of-life care. This chapter covers the four elements of communication – medical providers (especially physicians), patients and their families, the message, and the environment – in order to maintain patient dignity and compassionate palliative care.

The concept of dignity involves a perception of a sense of worth, honor, and respect that a person feels from others. It is an affirmation that the person exists and is not merely a checklist. The concept of dignity goes hand in hand with person-centered care by developing an interpersonal relationship that can iden-tify the needs of the patient and family, which then can enhance the expecta-tions of healing. Certain features have been identified as contributing to the concept of dignity, including respect, autonomy, empowerment, and commu-nication (Kennedy, 2016).

Patients with advanced diseases have to make medical decisions in the midst of intense physical and emotional distress. Having information regarding treat-ment options and prognosis is vital for patient decision-making. When infor-mation is delivered sensitively and appropriately, it can have a positive impact on a patient's emotions and promote reassurance. Information preferences vary among patients and in their disease trajectory – hence the need to tailor the timing, amount, and quality of information based on the patient's needs and situation.

We can identify four components of patient–physician communication, par-ticularly at end of life: the physician, the patient, the message, and the environ-ment (Table 10.1). Although each component can be viewed distinctly, they are oftentimes interconnected and are critical to the success of the communica-tion. Successful communication may involve verbal and nonverbal methods and may contribute to maintaining a person's sense of dignity. The purpose of this chapter is to discuss different factors that influence the physician's comfort

Table 10.1 Elements of Physician–Patient Communication at End of Life.

Physician

- Knowledge and expertise
- Psychological factors
- Comfort in communicating difficult information
- Perception of what patient knows, wants, and fears

Patient

- Question prompt sheets
- Standardized assessment tools
- Decisional control and information preferences
- Physician access

Message

- Manner of delivery
- Content of message
- Non-verbal aspects of care
- Follow-up

Environment

- Space
- Time
- Setting
- Technology

and experience in difficult conversations, evaluate patient factors that influence their communication and information preferences, explore the roles of the content and manner of how a message is delivered and its effect on patient perception of the physician, discuss the role of the setting and environment where communication is conducted, and, overall, highlight clinical interventions at bedside with potential to improve and restore dignity of patient and families.

The Physician

Despite evidence in the literature that early end-of-life care discussions with patients who have life-threatening conditions are highly beneficial and promote the likelihood of receiving care in concordance with their wishes, physicians often have difficulty conducting these discussions (Bruera, 2006; Fallowfield & Jenkins, 2004; Friedrichsen & Milberg, 2006). Factors cited in the literature that contribute to this difficulty include the fear of destroying hope and being perceived as less compassionate than others. Additionally, physicians might be concerned with provoking emotional distress not only to the patient but also themselves (Friedrichsen & Milberg, 2006; Russell & Ward, 2011; Meier & Back, 2001; Tanco et al., 2015). An attempt to balance emotions and confidence in their own diagnostic and prognostic abilities while trying to maintain the patient's trust and hope may contribute to the physician's sense of losing control (Friedrichsen & Milberg, 2006). Several of the emotions physicians feel may also be related to a change in the traditional role of healer to a "bearer of bad news." These may invoke various emotions of guilt that one did not do enough to cure the patient or alleviate their suffering.

As with the concept of person-centered care, having an established relationship with the patient allows the physician to identify nuances in a patient's care preferences as well as what that patient values and fears. This allows more familiarity and comfort with each other, particularly when delivering sensitive information. These conversations can often be quite challenging when the healthcare provider has not had a chance to establish a relationship with the patient and family yet.

A physician's confidence in their own knowledge base may affect their comfort in having difficult conversations with patients and their families. Within seconds, patients and families are able to access medical information, whether validated or not, through the internet. That information may consciously or subconsciously alter the expectations of the patient and family in the course of their disease. Physicians may feel challenged that they are unable to catch up with the influx of new data available and, at the same time, not sound dismissive of certain nonvalidated information.

Another factor in knowledge that affects communication is prognostication. Prognostication plays a key role in end-of-life choices. Having appropriate knowledge of prognostication is crucial in these discussions. However, physicians have been found to have a tendency to overestimate a patient's survival and may be able to predict better for patients who have a more immediate risk of dying (Glare et al., 2003). One process to curtail the challenge of prognosticating accurately is to have early advanced-care planning discussions. By individually adapting these discussions to the patient's hopes and goals and conducting them progressively through the patient's course of care, patients and families are empowered to express their personal preferences and goals; receive care concordant with their wishes; and have the opportunity to prepare physically, psychosocially, mentally, and financially for what awaits in their disease process (Agarwal & Epstein, 2018).

In the end, most physicians may simply just feel uncomfortable and unprepared to conduct end-of-life discussions. Trying to go through the literature may, at times, end up more confusing than helpful regarding how to conduct these conversations. Conveying the right balance of empathy and hope but not sounding overly effusive or bleak may be simpler taught than done. There are a variety of classes and strategies that explore empathic end-of-life communication, such as SPIKES (Baile et al., 2000) and Oncotalk (Back et al., 2007).

The Patient

Another strategy that has been found effective is the use of question prompt sheets. Question prompt sheets consist of structured questions that patients use to ask their healthcare team. Implementing a question prompt sheet has been shown to be beneficial for patient–physician communication while not prolonging clinic encounters (Arthur et al., 2017; Clayton et al., 2007). Arthur et al. were able to develop a single-page prompt sheet that incorporated relevant aspects of palliative care for patients attending an outpatient palliative care clinic; interestingly, they discovered that patients valued questions regarding end-of-life topics (Arthur et al., 2017). Furthermore, by utilizing a prompt sheet that can be used by both patients and caregivers, this allowed caregivers to feel involved and not isolated from the patient's care.

Although a prompt sheet allows patients chances to ask various questions that normally they would not have thought about or have the opportunity to ask, utilizing standardized assessment tools provides them a way to express their symptoms in an organized and systematic way. This allows the physician to evaluate the total physical and psychosocial symptomatology of a patient, including symptoms that may be missed due to limitations in time or when a patient is simply attempting to minimize their symptoms not to be a burden to the physician or their family. A frequently used assessment tool that measures a variety of common symptoms, particularly in palliative care patients, is the Edmonton Symptom Assessment System (ESAS) (Bruera, Kuehn, Miller, Selmser, & Macmillan, 1991).

Despite having a variety of methods available for patients to use to communicate their concerns to the physician, these can only be effective if physicians are able to access the patients and their families. There is a trend for care to be delivered more in the outpatient and home settings than in the hospital. Telephone-based intervention programs allow patients earlier access to care and symptom management, particularly in patients with significant debility, financial constraints, or logistic difficulties (Pimentel et al., 2015). These programs can be utilized to manage not only physical symptoms but also counseling needs.

Understanding a patient's decisional control preferences can facilitate patient satisfaction and improve quality of care. A patient's decision control preference may be either active, with the preference to make decisions by themselves; passive, with the preference of others making decisions for them; or shared, which is collective decision-making between patient and family and/or physician. Yennurajalingam et al. conducted a study over 11 countries and discovered that a majority of advanced cancer patients preferred active or shared decision-making (Yennurajalingam et al., 2018b). In another study conducted by their group, advanced cancer patients who had an accurate perception of their curability were noted to prefer a passive decision control preference (Yennurajalingam et al., 2018a). They found this consistent with previous studies that demonstrated patients preferring a more passive decisional approach with progression of their disease (Butow, Maclean, Dunn, Tattersall, & Boyer, 1997).

Information preferences regarding treatment and prognosis, how to receive the information, and the evaluation of physician communication and interpersonal skills can vary among patients (Innes & Payne, 2009). Let us take hope as an example. We mentioned that the fear of destroying hope may be one of the factors that contribute to physicians' difficulties in end-of-life communication. Hope is consistently mentioned as important to a patient but may have different meanings for each person. For example, patients favor ending a bad-news conversation with hopeful statements. They also often express a need for hope, even against all odds (Schofield, Carey, Love, Nehill, & Wein, 2006). At the same time, patients often hope for attainable goals such as optimal comfort in the remaining time and not necessarily unrealistic expectations (Van Vliet et al., 2013). On the other hand, some patients express the need to receive realistic information even if less optimistic (Parker et al., 2007). Some people argue that realistic information may nurture hope, while others argue that it destroys hope (Van Vliet et al., 2013).

The Message

The content and the manner in which information is delivered play a key role in how a patient receives the information and how he or she processes it. Physicians should be able to deliver the information in a way that does not omit important details and is understandable and at the same time does not aggravate the discomfort surrounding it. Knowing what the patients or family members understand about the illness is a good place to start. Having an established relationship with the patients and families helps in identifying what the patient knows and values. Moreover, incorporating a warning shot before bad news is delivered may help reduce the blow from the news (Ptacek & Eberhardt, 1996). Thereafter, physicians should be prepared that there may be various reactions after news is delivered. This is an opportunity to further explore patient and family reactions and allow them to express further any concerns and emotions. By doing these, a method to identify further patient and family needs is established, and a framework for patients to be able to trust and express their fears and concerns to the physician is developed.

Information must be delivered in an empathic and respectful way. There are mixed opinions about the use of metaphors and euphemisms when explaining things (Klein & Klein, 1987; Maguire & Faulkner, 1988). Some believe that language should be kept simple and straightforward, while others argue that euphemisms may help identify how much information the patient wants to know about their condition. After receiving the news, patients and families may have difficulty remembering the information presented, which can heighten anxiety and stress. Summarizing and regular probing by the physician of patients and families to gauge their understanding is recommended. Recording the conversation by written notes or audio recording also allows the physician to solve this problem, as well as allowing the patient an opportunity to relay the information discussed to family who were not present in the visit (Ptacek & Eberhardt, 1996; Fallowfield, 1993).

Nonverbal aspects of communication can also play a role in the patient's perception of their communication with the physician. Demonstrating active listening skills can convey empathy and involve demonstrating interest through actions such as head nodding, eye contact, timely responses, and summarizing what the patient discussed. A physician's posture can also affect a patient's perception of the physician's compassion. Patients preferred, and felt to be more compassionate, physicians who were sitting as compared to standing (Bruera et al., 2007; Strasser et al., 2005). Furthermore, physicians who were sitting were also felt to spend more time with the patient (Strasser et al., 2005). On the other hand, other factors, such as time spent on visit, warmth, patience, respect, and a caring attitude, were rated higher by patients as compared to physician posture (Bruera et al., 2007).

A regular component of every patient visit is the physical examination. However, with continued progression of modern technological machines, the reliance on physical examination for diagnostic purposes has decreased. Kadakia et al. described pragmatic and spiritual benefits that this routine and often-overlooked practice can provide (Kadakia et al., 2014). Patients described that the simple act of being examined can provide reassurance and validate their distress.

Interestingly, the content of the message may be found to be even more important than the manner it was delivered (Brown, Parker, Furber, & Thomas, 2011). Patients rely on information regarding their treatment options and prognosis to plan their future (Innes & Payne, 2009). However, as we have discussed, it is a challenge in delivering information that is both realistic and that does not destroy hope. In video-based studies conducted in an outpatient supportive care center, physicians delivering a less optimistic message were perceived to be less compassionate, trustworthy, and able to provide care (Tanco et al., 2015). Furthermore, when presented with a clinical scenario of continued patient decline, physicians who delivered either a more or less optimistic message were both found to have a worse overall impression. After knowing of the clinical decline, patients also rated physicians who delivered a more optimistic message to be less preferred for themselves and their families (Tanco et al., 2018). On the contrary, in a separate study, adult advanced cancer patients who received prognostic discussions from their oncologists were found to have a more favorable relationship with their physician three months after the prognostic discussion (Fenton et al., 2018).

What do physicians tell the patients, then? Should they deliver a realistic message that has the risk of the patients perceiving them as less compassionate, or should physicians trust that the patients will eventually appreciate their honesty and appreciate them better in the near future? The answer may be more than a single aspect at a single point in time. A combination of an empathic approach, nonverbal techniques, and development of trust through a relationship of care established earlier in the disease process may all contribute to a successful communication that focuses on the patient as the center of care and maintains their sense of dignity. Periodic pauses during the conversation allow information to settle in with the patient and family, as well as providing an opportunity to comfort them. This is also an opportunity to ask questions to gauge their understanding. It is not uncommon that patients and family may demonstrate episodes of denial or even anger (Fallowfield, 1993). In these moments, allowing them time and space to let their emotions flow and not confronting them is beneficial. At times, the conversation has to be conducted in multiple phases instead of one session. Frequent follow-ups via telephone or in person, particularly after difficult news has been delivered, should be done to follow up on any information that the patient and family would wish to clarify or information that they may have missed or not remembered or simply how they are coping with the news.

The Environment

All of these various techniques of communication must be delivered in an environment that allows the patient and family to know that they are the utmost priority at that moment. There should be enough space to accommodate all who are involved in the conversation, including the patient, family, and health-care providers. The use of video or phone conferencing may also allow family members who are not able to join physically to be a part of the discussions and prevent them from feeling excluded. At times, the patient may not wish to be involved in the conversation and prefer the family or a designated surrogate to make decisions for them. This should be clarified beforehand. The conversation should also be set at a time that is convenient for the patient and family as well as with enough time to allow them to absorb information, ask questions, and appropriately vent their emotions if needed (Ptacek & Eberhardt, 1996). In addition, the setting should be in a location where interruptions and noise are kept to a minimum. However, in a hospital setting, the noise level may be difficult to control. The presence of background music may help reduce distraction from hospital and clinic noise. Music has been used in different settings to help reduce stress and promote comfort (Zaza, Sellick, & Hillier, 2005; Kemper & McLean, 2008; Tansik & Routhieaux, 1999). Patients, caregivers, and healthcare providers found background music to be more pleasant and positive than ordinary hospital and clinic sounds (Perez-Cruz et al., 2012).

With improvement in technology, a focus on clinical efficiency, and the advent of electronic health records, computers have become a routine part of examination rooms. If used properly and strategically during the clinic visit to show relevant information such as imaging results, the use of the computer may be a powerful tool in communicating important information relevant to the patient's care and helping them understand further their current medical situation. However, when physicians are communicating to patients and families while working on the computer simultaneously to review medical records and type notes, this may result in detrimental effects in nonverbal communication.

The tactile noise from the frequent clicking of the keyboard and mouse, in addition to the decrease in eye contact as the physician spends more time looking at the computer, may contribute to a diminished sense of patient-centeredness. Furthermore, there is a risk that the physician may miss crucial psychosocial issues while trying to complete computer-related tasks when their attention is divided between the patient and the computer. Street et al. examined primary care providers' computer use during patient clinic visits and found that physicians who spent more time looking at the computer were rated to have poorer communication (Street et al., 2014). Additionally, in a study comparing the effect of the use of examination room computers on patient perception on physician compassion, communication skills, and professionalism, physicians who interacted with their patients face to face and not using the computer predominantly were perceived as more compassionate, professional, and communicating better than physicians who were using the examination room computer to access and enter information (Haider et al., 2018).

Conclusion

The elements identified in this chapter require leaders of medical academic institutions to make considerable investments in the structures and processes of end-of-life care. Structures and processes include settings that are not frequently available, such as supportive and palliative care centers and inpatient palliative care units with enough rooms with full beds, chairs, and space, as well as availability of interdisciplinary team members. Processes involve providing the time for these professionals to interact with the patient and family in an effective manner and also have the ability to follow up with patients and families during the process of end-of-life care. Only after the achievement of structural and procedural changes will communication outcomes be successfully implemented in healthcare facilities.

Discussion Questions

1. What role does patient–physician communication play at the end of life?
2. What are determining factors in patient–physician communication?
3. How does messaging affect patient–physician communication?

References

Agarwal, R., & Epstein, A. S. (2018). Advance care planning and end-of-life decision making for patients with cancer. *Seminars in Oncology Nursing* 34, 316–326.

Arthur, J., Yennu, S., Zapata, K. P., Cantu, H., Wu, J., Liu, D., & Bruera, E. (2017). Perception of helpfulness of a question prompt sheet among cancer patients attending outpatient palliative care. *Journal of Pain and Symptom Management* 53, 124–130.e1.

Back, A. L., Arnold, R. M., Baile, W. F., Fryer-Edwards, K. A., Alexander, S. C., Barley, G. E., . . . Tulsky, J. A. (2007). Efficacy of communication skills training for giving bad news and discussing transitions to palliative care. *Archives of Internal Medicine* 167(5), 453–460.

Baile, W. F., Buckman, R., Lenzi, R., Glober, G., Beale, E. A., & Kudelka, A. P. (2000). SPIKES – A six step protocol for delivering bad news: Application to the patient with cancer. *Oncologist* 5, 302–311.

Brown, V. A., Parker, P. A., Furber, L., & Thomas, A. L. (2011). Patient preferences for the delivery of bad news: The experience of a UK Cancer Centre. *European Journal of Cancer Care* 20, 56–61.

Bruera, E. (2006). Process and content of decision making by advanced cancer patients. *Journal of Clinical Oncology* 24, 1029–1030.

Bruera, E., Kuehn, N., Miller, M. J., Selmser, P., & Macmillan, K. (1991). The Edmonton Symptom Assessment System (ESAS): A simple method for the assessment of palliative care patients. *Journal of Palliative Care* 7, 6–9.

Bruera, E., Palmer, J. L., Pace, E., Zhang, K., Willey, J., Strasser, F., & Bennett, M. I. (2007). A randomized, controlled trial of physician postures when breaking bad news to cancer patients. *Palliative Medicine* 21, 501–505.

Butow, P. N., Maclean, M., Dunn, S. M., Tattersall, M. H., & Boyer, M. J. (1997). The dynamics of change: Cancer patients' preferences for information, involvement and support. *Annals of Oncology* 8, 857–863.

Clayton, J. M., Butow, P. N., Tattersall, M. H. N., Devine, R. J., Simpson, J. M., Aggarwal, G., . . . Noel, M. A. (2007). Randomized controlled trial of a prompt list to help advanced cancer patients and their caregivers to ask questions about prognosis and end-of-life care. *Journal of Clinical Oncology* 25, 715–723.

Fallowfield, L. (1993). Giving sad and bad news. *Lancet* 341, 476–478.

Fallowfield, L., & Jenkins, V. (2004). Communicating sad, bad, and difficult news in medicine. *Lancet* 363, 312–319.

Fenton, J. J., Duberstein, P. R., Kravitz, R. L., Xing, G., Tancredi, D. J., Fiscella, K., . . . Epstein, R. M. (2018). Impact of prognostic discussions on the patient–physician relationship: Prospective cohort study. *Journal of Clinical Oncology* 36, 225–230.

Friedrichsen, M., & Milberg, A. (2006). Concerns about losing control when breaking bad news to terminally ill patients with cancer: Physicians' perspective. *Journal of Palliative Medicine* 9, 673–682.

Glare, R., Virik, K., Jones, M., Hudson, M., Eychmuller, S., Simes, J., & Christakis, N. (2003). A systematic review of physicians' survival predictions in terminally ill cancer patients. *BMJ – British Medical Journal* 327, 195–198.

Haider, A., Tanco, K., Epner, M., Azhar, A., Williams, J., Liu, D. D., & Bruera, E. (2018). Physicians' compassion, communication skills, and professionalism with and without physicans' use of an examination room computer: A randomized clinical trial. *JAMA Oncology* 4, 879–881.

Innes, S., & Payne, S. (2009). Advanced cancer patients' prognostic information preferences: A review. *Palliative Medicine* 23, 29–39.

Kadakia, K. C., Hui, D., Chisholm, G. B., Frisbee-Hume, S. E., Williams, J. L., & Bruera, E. (2014). Cancer patients' perceptions regarding the value of the physical examination: A survey study. *Cancer* 120, 2215–2221.

Kemper, K. J., & McLean, T. W. (2008). Parents' attitudes and expectations about music's impact on pediatric oncology patients. *Journal of the Society for Integrative Oncology* 6, 146–149.

Kennedy, G. (2016). The importance of patient dignity in care at the end of life. *Ulster Medical Journal* 85, 45–48.

Klein, S., & Klein, R. (1987). Delivering bad news: The most challenging task in patient education. *Journal of the American Optometric Association* 58, 660–663.

Maguire, P., & Faulkner, A. (1988). Communicating with cancer patients: Handling bad news and difficult questions. *BMJ – British Medical Journal* 297, 907–909.

Meier, D. E., & Back, A. L. (2001). The inner life of physicians and care of the seriously ill. *JAMA – Journal of the American Medical Association* 286, 3007–3014.

Parker, S. M., Clayton, J. M., Hancock, K., Walder, S., Butow, P. N., Carrick, S., Currow, D., Ghersi, D., Glare, P., Hagerty, R., & Tattersall, M. H. (2007). A systematic review of prognostic/end-of-life communication with adults in the advanced stages of a life-limiting illness: Patient/caregiver preferences for the content, style, and timing of information. *Journal of Pain and Symptom Management* 34, 81–93.

Perez-Cruz, P., Nguyen, L., Rhondali, W., Hui, D., Palmer, J. L., Sevy, I., . . . Bruera, E. (2012). Attitudes and perceptions of patients, caregivers, and health care providers toward background music in patient care areas: An exploratory study. *Journal of Palliative Medicine* 15, 1130–1136.

Pimentel, L. E., Yennurajalingam, S., Chisholm, G., Edwards, T., Guerra-Sanchez, M., De La Cruz, M., . . . Bruera, E. (2015). The frequency and factors associated with the use of a dedicated supportive care center telephone triaging program in patients with advanced cancer at a comprehensive cancer center. *Journal of Pain and Symptom Management* 49, 939–944.

Ptacek, J. T., & Eberhardt, T. L. (1996). Breaking bad news. A review of the literature. *JAMA* 276, 496–502.

Russell, B. J., & Ward, A. M. (2011). Deciding what information is necessary: Do patients with advanced cancer want to know all the details? *Cancer Management and Research* 3, 191–199.

Schofield, P., Carey, M., Love, A., Nehill, C., & Wein, S. (2006). "Would you like to talk about your future treatment options?" Discussing the transition from curative cancer treatment to palliative care. *Palliative Medicine* 20, 397–406.

Strasser, F., Palmer, J. L., Willey, J., Shen, L., Shin, K., Sivesind, D., . . . Bruera, E. (2005). Impact of physician sitting versus standing during inpatient oncology consultations: Patients' preference and perception of compassion and duration: A randomized controlled trial. *Journal of Pain and Symptom Management* 29, 489–497.

Street, R. L. Jr., Liu, L., Farber, N. J., Chen, Y., Calvitti, A., Zuest, D., . . . Agha, Z. (2014). Provider interaction with the electronic health record: The effects on patient-centered communication in medical encounters. *Patient Education and Counseling* 96, 315–319.

Tanco, K., Azhar, A., Rhondali, W., Rodriguez-Nunez, A., Liu, D., Wu, J., . . . Bruera, E. (2018). The effect of message content and clinical outcome on patients' perception of physician compassion: A randomized controlled trial. *Oncologist* 23, 375–382.

Tanco, K., Rhondali, W., Perez-Cruz, P., Tanzi, S., Chisholm, G. B., Baile, W., . . . Bruera, E. (2015). Patient perception of physician compassion after a more optimistic vs a less optimistic message: A randomized controlled trial. *JAMA Oncology* 1, 176–183.

Tansik, D. A., & Routhieaux, R. (1999). Customer stress-relaxation: The impact of music in a hospital waiting room. *International Journal of Service Industry Management* 10, 68–81.

Van Vliet, L., Francke, A., Tomson, S., Plum, N., van der Wall, E., & Bensing, J. (2013). When cure is no option: How explicit and hopeful can information be given? A qualitative study in breast cancer. *Patient Education and Counseling* 90, 315–322.

Yennurajalingam, S., Lu, Z., Prado, B., Williams, J. L., Lim, K. H., & Bruera, E. (2018a). Association between advanced cancer patients' perception of curability and patients' characteristics, decisional control preferences, symptoms, and end-of-life quality care outcomes. *Journal of Palliative Medicine* 21, 1609–1616.

Yennurajalingam, S., Rodrigues, L. F., Shamieh, O. M., Tricou, C., Filbet, M., Naing, K., . . . Bruera, E. (2018b). Decisional control preferences among patients with advanced cancer: An international multicenter cross-sectional survey. *Palliative Medicine* 32, 870–880.

Zaza, C., Sellick, S. M., & Hillier, L. M. (2005). Coping with cancer: What do patients do. *Journal of Psychosocial Oncology* 23, 55–73.

Chapter 11

Holy Name Meditation

A Spiritual Intervention to Conserve the Dignity of Patients and Nurses

Jinsun Yong and Hun Lee

Although the physician-assisted suicide regulations have equated their programs with "dignity," this chapter refutes that correlation, insisting that dignity can more accurately be correlated with "spirituality." When the care of a patient is concerned with that patient's spirituality, dignity is ensured for both patient and caregiver. Testimonies from both palliative care providers as well as patients showed that a five-week meditation program encourages significant improvements in spiritual well-being and spiritual needs while resulting in reduced depression, anxiety, and burnout.

The Impact of the "Death With Dignity" Movement

On the first day of the year of 2019, Hawaii became the seventh state in the United States to legalize physician-assisted suicide. Modeled after Oregon's Death with Dignity Act, which took effect in 1997 to make Oregon the first state to legalize physician-assisted suicide, Hawaii's newly enacted Our Care, Our Choice Act allows terminally ill patients to take their lives with prescription drugs. This marks a victorious moment for advocacy groups like the Death with Dignity National Center, whose central tenet lies in the belief that "Death with dignity is about compassion, autonomy, and the right to choose."[1]

Identifying one's right to choose death as "death with dignity" has been a commonplace phenomenon in states and countries that seek to enact laws legalizing physician-assisted suicide.[2] Many advocates accordingly use the phrase "death with dignity" as a catchphrase for their cause, which has led many people to naturally equate the term with physician-assisted suicide. Such tendency has been increasingly prevalent in Asian countries, as illustrated by recent legislation addressing end-of-life care for terminally ill patients that begins with the following declaration:

The purpose of this Act is to prescribe matters necessary for life-sustaining treatment and determination to terminate, etc., life-sustaining treatment for patients in a hospice, receiving palliative care, and at the end of life, and the implementation thereof, and thereby to protect the *dignity* and value of human beings by assuring the best interests of the patients and by respecting their *self-determination*.

(Act on Decisions, 2017)

The first provision of the recently enacted Act on Decisions on Life-Sustaining Treatment for Patients in Hospice and Palliative Care or at the End of Life of South Korea, also known as the "Law on Well-Dying," reflects the Korean people's perception about what constitutes "death with dignity." The Korean media introduces the enactment of a law enabling patients and families to make decisions regarding the use of life-sustaining treatments as the acknowledgment of the right to die with *dignity*, revealing the people's tendency to equate dignity with the right to self-determination.

A Problematic Model: Dignity as Autonomy

The tenets of "death with dignity" movements pose a problem, however, since their understanding of dignity may easily undergird arguments for the likes of physician-assisted suicide and euthanasia. Indeed, increasingly more people in Korea are arguing for the legalization of physician-assisted suicide. They reason that this would ensure one's right to avoid suffering and choose one's own fate at the end-of-life stage. In other words, the right to self-choice is being touted as the key element of "death with dignity."

The idea of conserving one's dignity becomes an important issue when patients face a serious health problem like terminal illness. This is specifically why dignity has been historically linked to discussions on end-of-life decisions. Dignity is also inseparably related to spirituality, for the two are fundamental constructs of the human person. But when dignity is viewed apart from the spiritual dimension of personhood, it can lead to a reductionist understanding of dignity.

The current trend in Korea surrounding "death with dignity" is a good example of such a misconception. This idea illustrates how a partial understanding of dignity can be invoked as a fundamental principle in advocating for the right to hasten or even choose death. A more profound, holistic understanding of human existence, on the other hand, stands as a fundamental principle that argues against such views. In fact, attempts to conserve the dignity of palliative care patients by addressing their physical, psychological, social, and spiritual needs related to patient-defined dignity have shown that such interventions actually reduced their desire to hasten death (Chochinov et al., 2002).

Against this backdrop, the present chapter examines a more holistic view on dignity and thereby redefines "dignified death." The chapter then introduces an intervention that has shown positive effects in conserving and promoting such dignity for both patients and healthcare professionals.

A Holistic Understanding of Dignity

A number of authors summarize that the concept of human dignity originally stemmed from a religious standpoint that views man as God's image but was altered when the idea of dignity began to follow the Kantian emphasis on human reason (Barak, 2015; Cobb, Puchalski, & Rumbold, 2012). The former perspective encapsulates the concept of "inherent" or "intrinsic" dignity (also called "basic" dignity), which can be understood as "dignity we have on the basis of our shared humanity" (McCrudden, 2013). The idea that man is created in the image of God corresponds to a more holistic view of personhood that encompasses the physical, psychological, social, and spiritual dimensions of humanity. In the post-Kantian understanding of dignity, on the other hand, dignity tends to be ascribed to individuals with rational capacity. This view is summed up in the term "personal dignity," which emphasizes individual autonomy and personal choice as essential elements of personhood.

The subtly disparate views on dignity help explain how dignity language is used by both sides of the debate regarding euthanasia. Proponents of euthanasia tend to argue for the sake of "dignity as liberty," whereas those in opposition rely on the idea of "dignity as life" (McCrudden, 2013). Likewise, personal dignity has often been a fundamental principle in advocacy for the right to hasten death on one hand while being invoked as a basic principle to forbid hastened death on the other (Cobb et al., 2012). While the debate between two distinct conceptions of dignity continues, one thing seems certain: for terminally ill patients who ask for physician-assisted suicide, such a request is often associated with "fear of indignity" (McCrudden, 2013).

It is in this vein that dignity has been related to spirituality, for spirituality has been presented as significantly enhancing patients' overall quality of life. Although the definitions of spirituality do not mention dignity in the strictest sense, it has been widely accepted that "spirituality has to do with the inherent value and dignity of all persons, regardless of their health status" (Cobb et al., 2012). Empirical studies have demonstrated that spiritual meaning is positively correlated to the conservation of dignity among end-of-life patients (Chochinov et al., 2009) and that nurses prefer spiritual care as means to conserve dignity among terminally ill patients (Doorenbos, Wilson, Coenen, & Borse, 2006). In short, it may be said that enhancing spirituality and conserving dignity are directly related in the context of caring for those who fear *in*dignity in the face of death.

Spiritual Intervention to Conserve Dignity

It is in this context that my interdisciplinary research team has been working to develop and apply spiritual interventions to conserve the dignity of both healthcare professionals and their patients. Together with a number of oncology unit manager nurses at the Seoul St. Mary's Hospital who wished to provide quality spiritual care to their patients, my team developed what came to be known as the Spiritual Care Leadership Program (SCLP). Our primary goal was to transform the clinical setting into a "forest of healing" by fostering the individual trees (i.e., the healthcare professionals) who constitute the forest. To this end, the team developed the Holy Name Meditation Program to enhance the nurse leaders' quality of life, thereby increasing the quality of their care and eventually creating a healing work environment.

Dignity-Conserving Self-Care for Healthcare Professionals

The Holy Name Meditation Program was thus initially developed for middle-manager nurses. It was primarily based on Eknath Easwaran's (2008) Eight Point Program (EPP), a variation of which showed significant effects through numerous empirical studies in the United States. The central element of this program focused on the repetition of a Holy Word or Holy Name, which is a word or a phrase that one finds meaningful. This spiritual practice has been used since ancient times and is derived from various spiritual and religious traditions. It can be practiced easily and simply – as part of the routine day-to-day activities of life – at any time and in any place. It can thus be practiced by anyone, regardless of whether the individual has any religious beliefs or practices (Yong, Kim, Park, Seo, & Swinton, 2011).[3]

Our team was able to demonstrate and publish the numerous positive effects of the Holy Name Meditation Program on nurse leaders/managers, preceptors (Ra, 2011), young nurses (Seo, Yong, Park, & Kim, 2014), nursing students (Kang & Yong, 2019), and multidisciplinary groups. After five weeks of the Holy Name Meditation Program, which included five 90-minute sessions, middle-manager nurses in the experimental group showed significant improvements in spiritual well-being, spiritual integrity, and leadership practice while reporting reduced burnout compared to the control group (Yong et al., 2011). In a six-month follow-up, the experimental group showed significant improvements in spiritual well-being, spiritual needs, job satisfaction, and self-efficacy while demonstrating reduced depression, anxiety, and burnout (Yong et al., 2019). The results strongly suggest that the Holy Name Meditation Program can have long-term positive effects on nurse leaders' psychosocial and spiritual well-being.

It has been suggested that the wide array of spiritual interventions may be categorized into (1) therapeutic communication techniques, (2) therapy, and (3) self-care (Puchalski et al., 2009). The Holy Name Meditation Program is a form of meditation under the category of self-care, through which healthcare professionals can effectively enhance their quality of life and maintain their dignity amid a highly stressful, at times dehumanizing, work environment.

This can be seen from the following words from a nurse who participated in the Holy Name Meditation Program:

> When I work, I often find myself becoming angry, nervous, hesitant, or impatient without realizing it. I sometimes feel resentment against the people I meet when I am overwhelmed by so many tasks and requests. When a patient doesn't get better no matter how hard I try and provide the best care I can give, all my efforts seem meaningless, making me feel like a failure. When I feel that my colleagues are not helping me out while I am carrying the entire burden, it is difficult to control my mind and emotions. But once I started participating in the Spiritual Care Leadership Program and practicing the Holy Name Meditation as often as I could, I was able to organize my thoughts and reflect on myself. In the past, I always tried to blame others without looking deeply into myself. But now, I am able to step back and look around myself. I started to put myself into other people's shoes, trying to think and see from the perspectives of my patients and colleagues. I let go of my resentments and replaced them with forgiveness and consolation. This brought peace to my heart, and enabled me to control myself better in my everyday practice. There are probably many people out there who have doubted their profession. Is this really for me? There can be times when they want to give up or run away from their present reality. I may be one of them. However, I now realize that the nursing profession addresses human life, which is truly *dignified*. Hence, the profession requires a sincere heart and the special awareness that one has been called to perform a dignified task. The Holy Name Meditation constantly reminds me of this truth, and guides me to carry out my duties with a sincere heart. I will definitely try to continue my Holy Name Meditation practice even after the program, so that I can live a more hopeful and joyous life.
>
> (Department of Nursing, 2011)

Dignity-Conserving Therapeutic Communication Techniques

As a mode of self-care, the Holy Name Meditation can certainly enhance and conserve the dignity of healthcare professionals who practice it by enhancing their well-being. At the same time, Holy Name Meditation can help professionals develop therapeutic communication techniques (e.g., compassionate presence, listening) and thus nurture them to become better providers of spiritual care. Indeed, attributes such as compassion, caring, authenticity, and empathy of healthcare professionals have been identified as crucial qualities when it comes to promoting healing, wholeness, and wellness among patients who are seriously ill (Cobb et al., 2012, 288). By changing the attitude of healthcare professionals and transforming their behaviors, as well as implanting compassion and fostering dialogue skills, the Holy Name Meditation Program can dispose the intrinsic qualities of caregivers to provide dignity-conserving care to the patients they meet.

Dignity-Conserving Therapy for Cancer Patients

After verifying the Holy Name Meditation Program's positive effects on nurses, my research team developed an altered version of the program suitable for cancer patients. When provided directly to healthcare professionals, the Holy Name Meditation Program indirectly conserves the patients' dignity through the transformed qualities of the professionals themselves. But when provided directly to cancer patients, the Holy Name Meditation Program can directly impact the patients' dignity by improving their well-being.

This was demonstrated in a study that showed that five weeks of the Holy Name Meditation Program effectively improved cancer patients' spiritual well-being and significantly reduced their anxiety and depression (Yong et al., 2018). Given the trans-religious and easily self-applicable nature of the Holy Name Meditation, many cancer patients could practice it on their own to improve their quality of life and thus live a more dignified life despite their illness. The following testimony from a patient illustrates the healing effects of the intervention.

> *Colon cancer.* These simple words made my vision fuzzy, my body trembling all over, and my mind confused. I felt dejected about life and I was angry after I heard that I was diagnosed with colon cancer. Before I had colon cancer, I had to go to work early in the morning every day and it was certainly continuation of extreme fatigue and stress. I smoked two packs of cigarettes and drank ten cups of instant coffee all day long since early in the morning. Therefore, I had irregular eating habits and lack of sleeps. Now, I began to recite the Holy Name which is "Thank you, Lord" even though I could hardly think and mumble the phase because of treatment medications. I shouted inwardly whenever and wherever I could. As time went by, a change started in my body and my mind; I felt that anxiety, restlessness, and feelings of emptiness were decreased. As days went by, I sometimes wept uncontrollably when I recited the phase. As I repeated the phase of "Thank you, Lord," I actually began to pray for God. Through prayer, I have been experiencing many changes and receiving peace in my mind and blessing at the same time. As I prayed for giving thanks to God and tried to rid myself of greed, I found a peace of mind and I even thanked the Lord for the fact that I got cancer.
>
> (Gomez-Batiste & Connor, 2017)

Conclusion

In an increasingly technocratic world, people tend to believe that human beings can control everything, including one's life and death. This can be seen from people's desire to be able to decide when to die and their belief that the right to choose death and avoid suffering constitutes human dignity. The rise of spiritual care within the field of healthcare enables us to realize that this is not all there is to human dignity; if healthcare professionals can become compassionate caregivers who live a dignified life themselves, and if patients can receive therapies that enhance their sense of meaning and purpose in life, we can reduce ill people's desire for hastened death and enable them to meet their fate in peace. The Holy Name Meditation can be an efficacious means to provide this kind of dignity-conserving spiritual care for both healthcare professionals and patients, preparing us for the "good death" that has been described as follows.

> The ideal of the Good Death, as our ancestors defined it, was a natural death free of medical flailing. It did not require experts. It took place at home and was neither sudden nor lingering. Just as we do now, our ancestors hoped to die in a familiar place among close friends and family; to be safe and gently cared for in their hours of need; to have their last words heard and treasured; to express their love and forgiveness and to hear that they were loved and forgiven in turn. . . . Good Death was not necessarily painless or peaceful . . . it was an honest death. Nobody pretended that death was not in the room. A brave death, to our ancestors, was one of acceptance.
>
> (Butler, 2013)

Discussion Questions

1. How is the role of a palliative care nurse different from a non–palliative care nurse role?
2. How can spiritual intervention conserve dignity?

Notes

1. Taken from Sara Deskar, "Compassion, Autonomy, and the Right to Choose," from stories compiled and published on the Death with Dignity National Center's website. www.deathwithdignity.org/stories/sara-deskar-compassion-autonomy/.
2. For example, Washington state enacted the Washington Death with Dignity Act in 2008, and the District of Columbia enacted the D.C. Death with Dignity Act in 2016.
3. Note that in the 2011 study, the Holy Name Meditation Program was called the Spirituality Training Program.

References

Act on Decisions on Life-Sustaining Treatment for Patients in Hospice and Palliative Care or at the End of Life. (Enforcement Date 04. Aug, 2017.) Act No.14013, February 03, 2016, New Enactment, (S. Korea), n.1. Emphasis added.

Barak, A. (2015). *Human Dignity: The Constitutional Value and the Constitutional Right*, 6. Translated by D. Kayros. Cambridge: Cambridge University Press.

Butler, K. (2013). *Knocking on Heaven's Door*, 272–273. New York: Scribner.

Chochinov, H., Hack, T., Hassard, T., Kristjanson, L., McClement, S., & Harlos, M. (2002). Dignity in the terminally ill: A cross-sectional cohort study. *Lancet* 360, 2026–2030.

Chochinov, H., Hassard, T., McClement, S., Hack, T., Kristjanson, L., & Harlos, M. (2009). The landscape of distress in the terminally ill. *Journal of Pain Symptom and Management* 38(5), 641–649.

Cobb, M., Puchalski, C., & Rumbold, B. (Eds.). (2012). *The Oxford Textbook of Spirituality in Healthcare*, 145–146. Oxford: Oxford University Press.

Department of Nursing at Seoul St. Mary's Hospital. (2011). *Our Spiritual Care Leadership Journey*. Seoul, Korea.

Doorenbos, A., Wilson, S., Coenen, A., & Borse, N. (2006). Dignified dying: A phenomenon and actions among nurses in India. *International Nursing Review* 53, 28–33.

Easwaran, E. (2008). *Passage Meditation: Bringing the Deep Wisdom of the Heart into Daily Life*, 3rd ed. Tomales, CA: Nilgiri Press.

Gomez-Batiste, X., & Connor, S. (Eds.). (2017). *Building Integrated Palliative Care Programs and Services*, 338. Catalonia, Spain: Liberdúplex, Reprint.

Kang, S., & Yong, J. (2019). Effects of spirituality promotion program on spirituality, empathy, and perceived stress in nursing students. Paper presented at the Seventh Annual Meeting of the Spirituality and Heath, Welfare Society Conference. Seoul, Korea.

McCrudden, C. (Ed.). (2013). *Understanding Human Dignity*, 528–529. Oxford: Oxford University Press.

Puchalski, C., Virani, R., Baird, P., et al. (2009). Improving the quality of spiritual care as a dimension of palliative care: The report of the consensus conference. *Journal of Palliative Medicine* 12, 885–904.

Ra, J. (2011). Effects of a spiritually based training program on the spiritual and psychosocial well-being, and leadership of preceptor nurses. Unpublished PhD diss. The Catholic University of Korea, Seoul.

Seo, I., Yong, J., Park, J., & Kim, J. (2014). Spiritual and psychosocial effects of the spirituality promotion program on clinical nurses. *Journal of Korean Academy of Nursing* 44(6), 726–734.

Yong, J., Kim, J., Park, J., Seo, I., & Swinton, J. (2011). Effects of a spirituality training program on the spiritual and psychosocial well-being of hospital middle manager nurses in Korea. *Journal of Continuing Education in Nursing* 42, 280–288.

Yong, J., Park, J., Kim, J., Kim, P., Seo, I., & Lee, H. (2018). The effects of Holy Name Meditation on spiritual well-being, depression, and anxiety of patients with cancer. *Journal of Hospice & Palliative Nursing* 20(4), 368–376.

Yong, J., Park, J., Park, Y., Lee, H., Lee, G., & Rim, S. (2019). The effects of Holy Name Meditation on the quality of life of hospital middle manager nurses in Korea: 6 month follow-up. *Journal of Continuing Education in Nursing* (in progress).

Chapter 12

Disclosure of Diagnosis to Patients

The Casualty of Incomplete Health Setups for Palliative Care

Emmanuel Luyirika

Healthcare in Africa faces a number of challenges, especially with respect to palliative care. For many reasons, disclosing actual diagnoses to patients is problematic for both practitioners and families and can lead to future difficulties. This chapter explores some of these reasons.

Healthcare practice and provision in Africa are as diverse as the number of countries on the continent. Most of the countries in Africa have not attained the target of spending at least 15 percent of their national budgets on health, as they agreed in Article 25 of the Abuja Declaration (World Health Organization, 2011).

This underspending on health has resulted in poor development of not only health systems in general but also access to palliative care for life-limiting conditions such as HIV, cancer, other communicable and noncommunicable diseases, and aging per se. This is happening despite the fact that Africa is faced with a multiplicity of infectious and noncommunicable diseases afflicting the continent and a population that largely depends on out-of-pocket expenses to access health services, with the exception of a few countries such as Rwanda (Khokhar, 2017)

Because of the low spending on health, access to palliative care – including controlled medicines and radiotherapy – is still very poor on the continent, despite the various efforts that are largely spearheaded by nongovernmental organizations (NGOs) and faith-based organizations. Recent data from the Lancet Commission on access to palliative care and pain medicines indicate that Africa is one of the regions with the least access to these services. Many African countries import morphine equivalents that cover less than 1 percent of the national need. Hardly any African countries cover 65 percent of the national need for palliative care and opioids (Knaul et al., 2017).

Over 80 percent of patients with cancer present very late for any curative interventions to happen, and most of these patients would benefit from palliative care. Access to controlled medicines such as oral morphine and essential technologies such as radiotherapy are poorly distributed in the continent, with almost 25 countries having no access to radiotherapy (IAEA, 2013).

The low investment in health has not only affected access to medicines and radiotherapy but has also affected developing a sustainable manpower for service delivery, including palliative care. Where it has happened, the ability to deliver chronic and palliative care is grossly underdeveloped, and communication and disclosure of the diagnosis to patients is still poorly done. Nondisclosure or impartial disclosure of health conditions and prognosis to patients is a very common challenge within the context of palliative and end-of-life care. Many patients and their families often find themselves in situations where complete and effective communication and disclosure of the conditions they face is not achieved. This leaves them ignorant about the diagnosis and prognosis of their illnesses.

Barriers to Healthcare Communication

There are several factors that contribute to incomplete or ineffective communication between the health practitioner and patients faced with life-limiting illnesses.

Stigma

Stigma associated with the specific disease itself may become a barrier to truth telling. This dilemma was brought to the fore especially during the early days of the HIV epidemic and to an extent for other conditions such as cancer and mental illnesses. Telling a patient that they had HIV was complicated by the accompanying stigma and the implications for the spouse and the children, as well as the wider family from which the patient came. The stigma was even bigger than the death that the patients faced, and most of the energy by the families and health practitioners was spent on responding to the stigma rather than the needs of the patient. The stigma incapacitated both health practitioner and patient, and the communication of the truth became hard for both. This, in the end, compromised the options that the patient had access to and limited HIV prevention efforts for the patient's spouse and children, both born and unborn. In the context of cancer care, this delays access to definitive interventions and results in incurability of the disease.

Stigma of palliative and hospice care at the end of life is another issue within the professionals themselves and among the patients and families who would rather say they are managed by a physician or surgeon and not a palliative care or hospice specialist. Stigma plays a very serious roles in health disparities, too (Earnshaw & Quinn, 2011).

Age of the Patient

The situation around disclosure of the diagnosis and prognosis is even worse when the patient is a child below the age of consent. Many parents would not like to tell their children that they have a medical condition that may end in death. The parents find it difficult to cope with that reality, and even if they do cope, they may not want to be part of a team that tells it to their children. This creates a coalition of non–truth tellers involving the healthcare providers and the child's family. The risk is that children who have access to information may in the end start asking questions after they suspect. The earlier a child knows that the health providers and parents are telling the truth, the better – and discovering the lies breaks the trust between children and parents or providers. Evidence exists to show that children are as interested in being told about their conditions as adults are (Bikaako-Kajura et al., 2006).

Contextual Factors

There are several contextual factors that make this situation worse. These may be health practitioner or health system factors or may arise out of the patient's context.

The contextual factors for the health practitioner may include the culture in which the health practitioner was raised or is operating, the family situation, pressure and dynamics of the job, the professional upbringing and mentorship of the practitioner, and the legal and ethical framework and standards in the country of operation. The health practitioners may also not have a support system to offer patients all the possible diagnostic and treatment options, thereby limiting the amount of correct and reliable information they have access to in order to share with the patient.

For the patient, it may be their faith that hinders them from proceeding all the way to the diagnosis, inadequate access to resources, or the limited options of care available to them. Other factors include the lack of a support system for the health practitioner or the patient and the family's inability to cope with the diagnosis or prognosis. For some patients, especially in Africa, the systems, technology, and equipment for definitive diagnosis may not be present; this leaves health workers, patients, and their families with presumptive diagnoses.

Individual Patient and Health Provider Factors

Both the patient and health practitioner may have individual factors that hinder effective and successful communication and therefore truth telling at the end of life.

The health practitioner may also have individual factors that include a lack of communication skills, especially in breaking bad news and therefore to handle truth telling when patients with a life-limiting illness are in their care. At times they think that by not telling patients the truth, they are being helpful and protective of them. The health workers may also at times lack the support system to carry out that truth telling.

The level of education and therefore the ability of the patient and family to understand the medical concepts also play a role in way the health practitioner will be engaged and demand information.

Deaf and dumb patients, either as a pre-existing condition or as an acquired one, make it very complicated and affect effective communication and truth telling in palliative care at the end of life. This calls for skills that most health practitioners may not have. It is made worse if the system in which the service is being offered does not have experts for the deaf and dumb to support the palliative care teams.

Incomplete Palliative Care Teams

Successful delivery of palliative care and communication to the patient and family requires a complete multidisciplinary team of professionals to cover all aspects of patient care and communication. In many facilities, especially in Africa and parts of Asia, it is impossible to put teams together that include all required professionals, such as psychologists, counselors, social workers, and other allied health professionals because of the resource and system limitations. The few existing health providers get overwhelmed by patient numbers and hardly have enough time to spend with patients. Truth and complete communication become casualties.

Out-of-Pocket Payments for Services

According to the World Health Organization and World Bank, out-of-pocket costs for healthcare account for almost 45 percent of all healthcare costs in Africa and other low- and middle-income countries. Therefore, for many patients at the end of life, access to hospice and palliative care, where it exists, requires payment of fees. At that time, most patients in Africa who require palliative care do not have the health insurance, financial capacity, or money to pay for these services. This complicates the affordability at a time when the patient and family may not have the resources and are most vulnerable.

Poor Communication and Nondisclosure as a Serious Risk for Patients and Their Families

In some of the less-developed economies, such as in Africa, nondisclosure of the truth when a patient is facing a life-limiting illness exposes the patient and family to worsening of superstition and speculation, which further exposes them to exploitation by some of the nonconventional healers or "masqueraders" and the subsequent impoverishment as they seek nonexistent cures. There is also a risk of exposure of the patient to dangerous and futile remedies and procedures that may increase suffering at the end of life (Riechelmann, Krzyz-anowska, & Zimmerman, 2009).

In order to rise above all these risks, health practitioners in the context of palliative end-of-life care must maintain a high degree of integrity and must communicate with the patient and family appropriately to enable them to understand the diagnosis and prognosis with a view to helping them make the right decisions.

Failure by the healthcare system to create a culture where patients are told the truth professionally creates more suffering and loss of trust in health practitioners and the health system. It also exposes patients and their families to untold suffering and very often to unnecessary expenditure on remedies that are of no use or that are dangerous.

When patients and their families do not know the exact conditions they are suffering from, they are faced with questions and start wondering whether these conditions are treatable or curable. In addition, if no informative interaction happens with health workers, key decisions such as writing wills and preparation for the care of the children when a parent is dead are delayed or even neglected. This creates a very difficult situation for the children who are exploited when the mother or father is dead, especially in countries where legal and child protection systems are weak. If it is the man who is affected and dies without proper will writing and setting up teams of legal trustees, the widow and the children are often disenfranchised by greedy relatives and expensive and/or corrupt legal systems. Health workers do not often imagine that their failure to properly disclose the diagnosis and support the patient and prepare that patient's family for the eventualities may well exacerbate some sociocultural and legal complications.

Conclusion

Several research studies have demonstrated the importance that patients and their families attach to knowing the actual diagnosis and prognosis when faced with a life-limiting problem and what steps need to be taken to cure it, ameliorate it, or cope with it. This is irrespective of whether the patient is a child or an adult (Bikaako-Kajura et al., 2006).

As universal health coverage schemes are being designed and implemented in Africa and the rest of the world, emphasis should be put on providing frameworks that include palliative care. Such frameworks should also strengthen the health infrastructure that supports developing and entrenching patient-centered communication skills for health providers.

Discussion Questions

1. How can one offer quality end-of-life care with minimal-quality health-care infrastructure?

2. Though the author recognizes that there are limited resources available in healthcare infrastructure, can you agree that palliative care still can be achieved in a minimal-quality healthcare infrastructure?

References

Bikaako-Kajura, W., Luyirika, E., Purcel, D. W., Downing, J., Kaharuza, F., Mermin, J., . . . Bunnell, R. (2006). Disclosure of HIV status and adherence to daily drug regimens among HIV-infected children in Uganda. *AIDS Behaviour* 10(4 Suppl.), S85–93.

Earnshaw, V. A., & Quinn, D. M. (2011). The impact of stigma in healthcare on people living with chronic illnesses. *Journal of Health Psychology* 17(2), 157–168. doi:10.1177/1359105311414952.

IAEA. (2013). Radiotherapy coverage worldwide. www.iaea.org/sites/default/files/18/03/pact-radiotherapy-coverage-010114.pdf.

Khokhar, T. (2017). Out-of-pocket health expenses; 100 million people pushed into poverty by health costs in 2010. https://blogs.worldbank.org/opendata/chart-100-million-people-pushed-poverty-health-costs-2010.

Knaul, F. M., Farmer, P. E., Krakauer, E. L., De Lima, L., Bhadelia, A., Kwete, X. J., . . . Rajagopal, M. R. (2017). Alleviating the access abyss in palliative care and pain relief – an imperative of universal health coverage. *Lancet* 391(10128).

Riechelmann, R., Krzyzanowska, M. K., & Zimmermann, C. (2009). Futile medication use in terminally ill cancer patients. *Support Care Cancer* 17(6), 745–748. doi:10.1007/s00520-008-0541-y.

World Health Organization. (2011). *The Abuja Declaration: Ten Years On.* Geneva: World Health Organization, 53.

Part 3

New Direction on Palliative Care

Chapter 13

Challenges to Dignity From Medically Assisted Death

Lessons From Canada

Sister Nuala Patricia Kenny

Dignity is a complex concept with many meanings in theology, philosophy, and politics, but it is far more than an esoteric notion to be pulled out of a language grab bag with reference to death. Dignity is not autonomous and is not the same as a "good death." Because human beings are made in the image of God, they share a God-given dignity – which cannot be lost in weakness, in undignified situations, or in dying. Being a patient in a health-care context is to be in a situation of need, dependence, and vulnerability – which can threaten a person's sense of dignity. In addition, life stories of physical, emotional, and sexual abuse, poverty, and social marginalization uncover constant threats to a sense of dignity. As Christians, however, we do not seek suffering; we have a duty to relieve it where possible but believe that through our pain and suffering, we can share in the redemptive work of Christ.

This book examines the notion of dignity in international healthcare contexts, with specific attention to serious and terminal illness and the role of palliative care. The role of "death with dignity" in the unique experience of Canada's legalization of medically assisted death (MAD) provides many lessons for those in countries that have legalized medically assisted death and those con-templating it.

These lessons include the need to recognize different understandings of dig-nity and the role of autonomy in contemporary bioethics; the power of media, language, and medically assisted death activists; the experience of dignity and its loss in illness, disease, disability, and dying; and the influence of belief in biotechnology to deliver us from all our suffering in secular societies. There were also lessons regarding confusion for many Catholics regarding Church teaching regarding medical decisions, especially for serious illness and dying, and the purpose and goals of end-of-life palliative care.

A chosen and controlled death has rapidly become the new normal for a "good death," and the majority of Catholics see no problem with it. Because of the significance of the faith dimension and spiritual focus, there are serious challenges for evangelization and catechesis. Throughout salvation history, prophets have been called forth to confront particular situations contrary to the reign of a loving and merciful God (Bruggemann, 2001). Today, the legalization of medically assisted death cries out for prophetic resistance to this dangerous understanding of "death with dignity" and prophetic witness to care and compassion.

Medically Assisted Death and the Canadian Experience

On February 6, 2015, the Supreme Court of Canada (SCC), in a stunningly broad decision, struck down Criminal Code prohibitions against medically assisted death for competent adults who have a grievous and irremediable medical condition (including an illness, disease, or disability) that causes enduring suffering that is intolerable to them (*Carter v Canada*, 2015). The decision was not confined to terminal illness or dying and assured protection of the vulnerable and of conscience. It was unique in that it was not confined to terminal illness or dying; it decriminalized both medically assisted suicide and physician-performed euthanasia and was the result not of legislation but of a rare, unanimous Supreme Court of Canada decision that affected the entire country. In the decision, the notion of dignity in the case was directly tied to autonomy, rational choice, and control. The challenge to the legal prohibition against assisted suicide and euthanasia was based on a Canadian Charter of Rights and Freedoms argument. Because this was a court decision, a 16-month stay, June 2016, Bill C-14 regulating Medical Aid in Dying (MAID) came into effect in Canada. It has been rapidly normalized as *the* good death and cries out for rediscovering the art of dying in our time (Kenny, 2017).

The 2015 Supreme Court decision was the result of a long history with two features: legislative and legal activity and media and special interest influence on public understanding and public discourse. In 1993, Sue Rodriguez submitted to the courts that section 241(b) of the Criminal Code, which prohibited assisted suicide, was constitutionally invalid. She suffered from amyotrophic lateral sclerosis (ALS), a rapidly progressive neurological disease, and wanted a physician's help in ending her own life at the time of her choosing. A 5–4 majority of the Supreme Court upheld the section. In international experience at that time, assisted suicide was legal in Switzerland and illegal, but not prosecuted, in the Netherlands.

Between 1993 and 2012, a number of federal legislative attempts to legalize assisted suicide failed. Proponents decided to pursue judicial remedy. So, in April 2012, the province of British Columbia's Civil Liberties Association filed on behalf of Gloria Taylor and Kay Carter. The two women also suffered from neurodegenerative diseases and wanted the right to have a doctor help them to die. This case was ultimately appealed to the Supreme Court and resulted in the February 6, 2015, SCC decision. By 2015, things had changed, and assisted suicide was legal in a number of countries in Western Europe and in Oregon, Washington, and Vermont.

From early notions of "mercy killing" to "the right to die" (and the right to oblige others to assist) and death with dignity, the corruption of language has been a major factor. Parallel with the formal strategies to legalize medically assisted suicide, the media has filled us with vivid images of persons dying in intractable pain requesting it. Modern medicine can do much to relieve pain and other serious symptoms. In fact, persons rarely request MAD because of pain but for psychological distress, uncertainty about future care needs, the desire to control death, fear of dependence, feelings of loss of dignity, fear of abandonment, guilt at being a burden to others, and loss of meaning (Emanuel, Fairclough, & Emanuel, 2000; Ganzini, Gay, & Dobscha, 2008). These are issues of deep human suffering.

Major advances in the power of medical technology in the past 50 years have created death-defying technology with the portable ventilator, cardiopulmonary resuscitation, cardiac defibrillators, and organ transplantation. These advances have occurred in increasingly secular societies (Carter, 1993). Technology and secularism combine to foster belief in the technology to save us from death and to cure all our ills (Fukuyama, 2002). Because there is no prescription or surgical procedure to eliminate suffering, a controlled, technically produced death has become the "treatment" (Cassell, 1991).

The Many Meanings of Dignity

As seen in the Sue Rodriguez case in Canada, dignity emerged as an explicit issue in healthcare ethics in the 1970s in discussions about dying and the right to "die with dignity." It was invoked by those who supported the legalization of medically assisted death and by those who opposed the intentional ending of another's life, even at their request, as an assault on human dignity (Sulmasy, 2002). There is widespread support for the notion that persons have a right to a dignified and humane dying and death. However, there are radically different understandings of what this means.

Dignity rapidly became central in debates surrounding the increasing power of science and technology in controlling human life, especially with emerging genetic, reproductive, and enhancement technologies; in research involving human subjects; and in health policy debates in aging societies. Respecting patient dignity also became an issue in medical education because of contemporary bioethics and the commercialization and commodification of healthcare. It became very clear that dignity is a complex concept with many meanings in theology, philosophy, and politics. However, it is far more than an esoteric and theoretical notion. The promotion and preservation of dignity are essential components in respectful and effective healthcare (Pellegrino, Schulman, & Merrill, 2009).

For some, equal dignity and respect are owed to all human life. No one can judge some lives "not worth living," even the person whose life is under consideration. Others believe that respect for the dignity and autonomy of all requires us to defer to personal choice. In other analyses, there is a conceptual distinction between dignity and autonomy, and dignity is prior to the value of autonomy. For many, human dignity rests on our higher mental capacities and rationality, with implications for some of the most vulnerable among us, including infants and children who will never have competence and persons with loss of cognitive capacity such as dementia.

Because of its centrality in the medically assisted death issue in Canada, a brief review of the "tangled sources" of human dignity in history can be helpful (Schulman, 2009).

Dignity did not enter the Western moral vocabulary or modern bioethics through the Judeo-Christian heritage. In ancient Greece and Rome, "dignus" and "dignitas" conveyed the notion of a rare excellence worthy of esteem as demonstrated in statesmanship, high achievement in athletic performance, and acts of heroism. These ancient notions invite judgments about distinctions where dignity is only for some. However, for the Stoics, humans have dignity because they possess reason and can choose to live in a thoughtful way.

In modern philosophy, Immanuel Kant has had profound influence, especially on modern bioethics. In Kantian moral philosophy, all humans possess dignity because of their rational autonomy and the shared human capacity to set our own goals and ends. Rational autonomy has been highlighted by most commentators. However, Byers has noted the importance of Kant's emphasis on the shared humanity of persons, which has implications for situations of dependence on others and inevitable vulnerability, such as in illness, dying, and the frailty of aging (Byers, 2016). Kant demands respect for all persons and forbids the use of another person for one's own ends. Unfortunately, his philosophy created a rigid distinction between duty/deontological analysis and consequential analysis of moral problems, which does not serve many moral issues well. He does not attend to other features of our humanity, including love, loyalty, and other emotions, and so has a narrow account of the moral life. If dignity is dependent on the rational will, what of those who do not yet have rational autonomy: infants, those with profound cognitive impairment who have never had rational autonomy, and those who have lost autonomy such as persons with dementia?

As modern bioethics develops in increasingly secular and pluralist societies, there is study of these philosophical concepts. In an early bioethics work, Beyleveld and Brownsword use dignity as empowerment, constraint on individual choices, and "dignified conduct" (2001). Kass states, "In sum, the human being has special dignity because he shares in the godlike powers of reason, freedom, judgment, and moral concern and, as a result, lives a life freighted with moral self-consciousness – a life above and beyond what other animals are capable of" (2002, 325). Meilander provides an excellent summary of the tension between the views of dignity. For some, dignity is a "floor" of basic respect and care. For others, it is a about excellence, setting a conflict between an ethic of equality vs an ethic of quality (2007). The essential difference still operative today is between intrinsic and extrinsic dignity. Intrinsic dignity cannot be gained or lost. It is about inherent worth. Extrinsic or attributed dignity is based on external measures such as social status, appearance, and so forth. It can be gained or lost by the opinion of others.

There is some important feminist philosophy work that critiques rigid understandings of autonomy and independence. It provides support for notions of interdependence of all persons and relational autonomy (Mackenie, Rogers, & Dodds, 2013).

Because of the differences in understanding dignity, Macklin claims that "appeals to dignity are either vague restatement of other, more precise, notions or mere slogans that add nothing to the understanding of the topic . . . a useless concept in medical ethics and can be eliminated without any loss of content" (2003). Dresser argues persuasively that Macklin's claim is unpersuasive for at least three reasons: claiming the concept is vague implies other bioethical concepts such as justice, fairness, and rights are not imprecise; those invoking dignity do not always give a full account, which is a reason to do more research, not to abandon the concept; and its lack of respect for those for whom dignity is an important concern that represents something over and above respect for autonomy (2009).

Religious claims about dignity exemplify the belief that dignity is distinct from autonomy. Gelernter, from the Jewish perspective, identifies the "irreducibly religious character of human dignity" (2009). Biblical religious understandings are rooted in the belief that human beings are made in the image of God and so share in a God-given dignity. Because dignity is an inherent quality of the children of God, it is not an attribute lost in weakness or in undignified situations. Dignity as a human person is rooted in our creation in the image and likeness of God: "So God created man in his own image, in the image of God he created him, male and female he created them" (Genesis 1:26–27). This belief calls us to see this image in all humans, even those broken and wounded in body, mind, or soul.

The Catholic Church teaches that "The dignity of man [sic] rests above all on the fact that he is called to communion with God" (*Catechism of the Catholic Church, no. 27*). The notion of dignity is central in Catholic social teaching, but there is little explication of dignity in recent encyclicals where one might expect it. They focus on threats to human dignity, especially from advances in technology. In *Evangelium Vitae* (1995),

> Every individual, precisely by the mystery of the Word of God who was made flesh is entrusted to the maternal care of the Church. Therefore every threat to human dignity and life must necessarily be felt in the Church's very heart; it cannot but affect her at the core of her faith in the redemptive

Incarnation of the Son of God, and engage her in her mission of proclaiming the Gospel of life in all the world, and to every creature.

The 2008 *Dignitatis Personae* spends little time on dignity, though it is pivotal:

God has created every human being in his own image, and his Son has made it possible for us to become children of God. By taking the interrelationship of these dimensions, the human and the divine, as the starting point, one understands better why it is that man has unassailable value: he possesses an eternal vocation and is called to share in the trinitarian love of the living God.

Dependence on religious beliefs regarding dignity is difficult for secular societies, but these beliefs can help us reflect on being human. Significantly, modern constitutions and declarations of rights, including the United Nations' *Universal Declaration of Human Rights* (1948), affirm belief in "the inherent and of the equal and inalienable rights of all members of the human family . . . the foundation of freedom, justice and peace in the world." Although human dignity is pivotal in these documents, the meaning and foundations are not defined. However, it is notable that these declarations were agreed upon by nations of differing religions, cultures, and histories.

Whether from classical philosophy, modern bioethics, or religious beliefs, theoretical understandings of dignity will guide whether and how we think about it in our care of sick and suffering persons.

The Experience of Dignity and Loss of Identity

Important as it is, theory about dignity is not the same thing as the personal experience of human dignity. Dignity is a lived reality. The notion of dignity overlaps with others such as pride, self-respect, well-being, worth, and self-esteem. In ordinary life, dignity is understood as something far more than just control and rational choice. Humans become aware of their own dignity when it is threatened. This occurs in major tragic situations such as war and genocide. A familiar and more general experience of awareness of threats to dignity occurs in healthcare. Being a patient in a healthcare context is to be in a situation of need, dependence, and vulnerability. Precisely because we are embodied humans with frailty and physical limitations and embedded in societies and systems of healthcare with interests and biases, a healthcare encounter brings theoretical issues into real lives.

The experience of loss of dignity is common in serious and chronic life-limiting illness and in dying. The Canadian experience learned quickly that one of the major reasons persons request medically assisted death is their sense of a loss of dignity in the experiences of serious illness and dying. So it is crucially important to explore the meaning and experience of dignity for patients coping with illness, dependence, and dying and the consequences of the sense of loss of dignity for whole-person care. We need to understand more deeply what persons mean when they experience a loss of dignity generally and in serious life-altering and life-threatening illness in particular. In serious illness and in dependence for care needs, loss of privacy; forced intimacy with strangers; and intrusion into the private areas of life, such as help with bathing and toileting, are guaranteed to be embarrassing and undignified experiences. When the medical condition causes disfigurement or exceptionally unpleasant and humiliating symptoms, such as incontinence, the empathic and respectful response of caregivers is essential. Restoration of dignity is a crucial goal of care. In fact, all care will be limited in its ability to provide comfort if this loss of dignity is not recognized and addressed. When dignity is conflated with autonomy, we can fail to recognize that bioethical concerns for autonomy, choice, and consent can be fully respected, yet the patient can still experience a sense of the loss of dignity.

These issues, and others unique to each person, will only be appreciated if we learn to attend to the patient's life story. Each patient's life story is utterly unique and will profoundly influence their illness experience (Kleinman, 1988). Over the past 20 years, medicine has come to recognize the difference between a case history and an illness narrative (Hunter, 1993). The medical case history is a unique genre. It is used in medicine to obtain a detailed and highly structured account of the patient's "presenting complaint," the history of the illness and features that have made the symptoms worse or better and family history of disease. The case history is directed to the diagnosis of the underlying pathology – illness, disease, or disability – causing the symptoms. Historically, it taught medical trainees to rigidly exclude factors considered irrelevant to the medical diagnosis. As Western medicine became more attentive to the importance of emotional, socioeconomic, spiritual, and cultural determinants of health and healing in "whole-person care," these personal factors have been included in a social component of the case history. Just as meticulous attention to the mechanics of consent and informed choice will not eliminate all threats to dignity, so too focused attention on the facts of a social history cannot reveal threats from the unique life story of a patient.

Illness narratives in autobiography, biography, and blog can help us understand these deeper issues. The power of stories in opening up conversations on the issues and dilemmas in modern healthcare, especially in terminal illness and dying, has been shown in the enormous popularity of Gawande's *Being Mortal: Medicine and What Matters in the End* (2014).

Over a lifetime, dignity and worth can be honored and promoted or compromised and eroded. Those who come to healthcare crises with a healthy, unbroken sense of their inherent dignity and personal worth can experience the indignity of illness and dependence. For others, their often-undignified life experiences have deformed or crushed any sense of personal dignity. Life stories of physical, emotional, and sexual abuse; poverty; and social marginalization uncover constant threats to a sense of dignity, making them highly vulnerable to further erosion of a sense of worth and sense of having lost their place in the human community.

Loss of identity in illness is intimately connected to a sense of loss of dignity. Identity is who we know ourselves to be; it is complex and ineffable, even sacred. Being literally and figuratively captured, constrained, and changed by physical and emotional pain challenges our identity in profound ways. Our physical appearance and strength can be profoundly altered; the talents and abilities that defined us and in which we took pride can be irretrievably lost; our role in our families, work, and our communities might be unalterably compromised. We can feel that we are truly falling apart and painfully experience a very real identity crisis.

Dementia raises a new awareness of the deep mystery of personal identity. Some, trying to provide consolation to loved ones in the face of the cognitive decline, failure of recognition, behavioral changes, and paranoia in dementia, say to the family, "She is not the person she once was." Far from consoling them, this kind of thinking adds to their suffering. Our culture insists that the human person is defined by rationality, autonomy, and choice. Dementia has assumed a special status in our time, embodying as it does weakness, dependence, indignity, irrationality, and loss of identity. There are ongoing philosophical debates regarding our identity as persons. Some have a falsely dualistic anthropology that distinguishes human beings from human persons. Some believe that those who have lost their cognitive capacities are nonpersons, raising many deep ethical issues. These beliefs put those with dementia at great risk, particularly with the legalization of medically assisted death.

I have called you by your name, you are mine (Isaiah 43:1).

For Christians, our identity as persons is, like dignity, an ontological, essential concept. It is not a functional concept to be lost when our capacities fail. Christian belief in our interdependence as children of God and the importance of communion and community challenges us to accept the deep relational challenges of respect and care for those with dementia and all cognitive decline.

Vulnerability

Vulnerability is generally understood as the state of being exposed to the possibility of being harmed physically or emotionally. Vulnerability is neither exceptional nor optional in the human condition. It is an inevitable in the fact of our being both embedded in families and communities and embodied in flesh and bone. Mackenie and colleagues (2013) propose that vulnerability may be inherent in this embedded and embodied human state, situational and caused or exacerbated by specific acute or chronic conditions, including personal, health status, socioeconomic factors, and the environment, or caused by unique pathogenic factors in personal history. A history of brokenness and marginalization, both self-imposed and socially isolated, brings a special form of this pathologic vulnerability. Autonomy, rights, and choice are so highly valorized today that there can be failure to recognize how they are affected adversely by inherent vulnerability, environments of care, and perpetuation of vulnerability in public policies and professional practices (Matthews & Tobin, 2016).

Work on vulnerability and resilience has also explored the notions of discretionary vulnerability, which arises as a result of deliberate decisions by persons themselves or from third parties such as the court (Lotz, 2016). A particular aspect in the healthcare context arises when we need to trust healthcare professionals and deliberately place ourselves in a situation of vulnerability. Doctors and other professionals are themselves challenged to reject the commercialization and commodification of healthcare and hold to that moral core of medicine, which is necessary to recognize vulnerability and respect the dignity of all patients (Pellegrino & Thomasma, 1988).

Some raise concerns raised regarding a focus on vulnerability because it can be paternalistic and oppressive. It can extend social control, and labeling persons and groups as vulnerable can result in stigma and marginalization rather than their empowerment and protection (Brown, 2011).

How the Spiritual Focus Changes the Interpretation of the Medical Outcome

Precisely because of the vulnerability in illness, a healthcare encounter for ourselves and our loved ones is a time and place of spiritual and moral meaning. Uncertainty, dependence, lack of control, and fear for the future provoke deep questions of meaning, even for the most secular among us.

Jesus's ministry of healing and reconciliation shaped and focused the moral and spiritual meaning for Christians. In his ministry of healing, Jesus's responses to the sick and suffering were characterized by attention to and cure of the physical. He also healed their emotional distress and restored a sense of integrity from the disintegration of dependence and serious illness and returned the often isolated and feared sick person to the community. The woman with the hemorrhage who suffered a humiliating condition and was ritually unclean so she could not enter the temple to pray is a marvelous example. After long, painful, and unsuccessful treatments under many doctors, she comes to Jesus but does not consider herself worthy to even speak to him: "and she said to herself, 'If I can only touch his cloak I shall be well again.' Jesus turned round and saw her; and he said to her, 'Courage, your faith has restored you to health.' And from that moment the woman was well again" (Matthew 9:20–22).

Although there is no scriptural basis for the three falls of Christ during His Passion, the traditional piety of the Stations of the Cross has intuitively recognized the threefold nature of human suffering: physical, psychological and emotional, and spiritual.

> For it is not as if we had a high priest who was incapable of feeling our weakness with us; but we have one who has been tempted in every way that we are, though he is without sin.
>
> (Hebrews 4:15)

During his Passion, Jesus experiences all of these forms of suffering in his scourging, abandonment, betrayal, loneliness, humiliation, seeing his loved ones suffer because he suffered, and seeing his lifework end as an apparent failure. Falling is a powerful analogy. In the split seconds of a fall, we experience a terrifying loss of control, and the consequences of a fall can be life altering. Pain and other physical symptoms, psychological and emotional distress, and spiritual suffering are distinct realities. Contemporary medicine's lack of attention to suffering can be traced to a worldview that separates mind and body while rejecting the notion of the spiritual.

There is no quick-fix medication or miracle of a procedure for spiritual suffering. As Pope John Paul II has said,

> Suffering is something which is *still wider* than sickness, more complex and at the same time still more deeply rooted in humanity itself. A certain idea of this problem comes from the distinction between physical suffering and moral suffering... *physical suffering* is present when "the body is hurting" in some way, whereas *moral suffering* is "pain of the soul."
>
> (*Salvifici Doloris*, 1984)

Suffering, the subject of much theological and philosophical thought, is a mystery, not in the sense of a puzzle to be solved but in the deeper sense of something not fully knowable. Suffering challenges us to drink the cup that Jesus drank and to find meaning that transforms the experience of our own personal suffering. Most human suffering occurs in situations where there is no physical disease or impairment. Just think of the anguish of a mother whose child is lost to drugs and prostitution or someone with survivor's guilt after a horrific disaster. Many who have serious illness, disabilities, and even those who are dying can experience no significant suffering because they are at peace. Suffering is not optional in human life, and it is irreducibly unique and particular to the person. However, some common dynamics of suffering have been identified, including a profound sense of loneliness, isolation and marginalization, an experience of a disintegration of mind and body, and a total loss of control and of "voice." All of these dynamics need to be taken into account in the care and support of those who suffer.

Jesus experienced physical abuse and was subjected to profound disrespect, degradation, and public humiliation during his way to the cross (Brown,

1994). The Jewish authorities mocked him for claiming to be a prophet. He also endured being spit upon in contempt and outrage for blasphemy. In the Old Testament, spitting is a degrading punishment for the guilty.

> The soldiers . . . dressed him up in purple, twisted some thorns into a crown and put it on him. And they began saluting him, 'Hail, king of the Jews!' They struck his head with a reed and spat on him; and they went down on their knees to do him homage. And when they had finished making fun of him, they took off the purple and dressed him in his own clothes.
> (Mark 15:1–20)

Jesus also experienced challenges to his identity. Since his time with the elders in the Jerusalem synagogue during the Passover of his 12th year and his reading from the prophet Isaiah regarding the blind seeing, the oppressed going free, and the good news to the poor being fulfilled in their sight, Jesus has a growing sense of who he is. This sense of identity is strengthened at his baptism by John in the Jordan: "No sooner had he come up out of the water than he saw the heavens torn apart and the Spirit, like a dove, descending on him. And a voice from heaven, 'You are my Son, the Beloved; my favor rests on you'" (Mark 1:9–11). This identity as Son of God was confirmed again at the Transfiguration: "And a cloud came, covering them in shadow; and there came a voice from the cloud, 'This is my Son, the Beloved. Listen to him'" (Mark 9:2–8).

So Jesus confidently calls God *Abba*, Father. Jesus has multitudes flocking after him to hear his message and be cured. He enters Jerusalem to the adulation of the crowds waving palm fronds and hailing him. But here, just a few days later, Jesus, the popular healer, the "well-beloved Son," is now a condemned criminal and an outcast. His identity, both who he is and his role in salvation history, is now challenged (Martin, 2014). And in some truly mysterious way, taking up the cross is essential to Jesus's identity: "Then Jesus said to his disciples, 'If anyone wants to be a follower of mine. Let him renounce himself and take up his cross and follow me. For anyone who wants to save his life will lose it; but anyone who loses his life for my sake will find it'" (Matthew 16:24–25).

Many persons today facing serious physical and cognitive illness can identify with Jesus's experience of indignity, humiliation, and loss of identity.

Religious coping is about how we make use of beliefs, practices, and community to make sense of and respond to tragedy and loss. Individuals are more likely to turn to religion in crisis if religion mattered in their life. In religious understanding, times of difficulty can be holy times because they bring us in touch with the mystery of life, and they force us to face limitations. They can also be dark nights of the soul. So, spiritual care is crucial in promoting the Christian understanding of suffering and in conserving dignity and identity in illness and dying (Lazenby, McCorkindale, & Sulmasy, 2014).

Preserving and Promoting Dignity for the Seriously Ill and Dying

Christians are called to prophetic resistance against the medicalization of human suffering and to find in Jesus's experience a source of meaning and strength for decisions in illness and dying. Now that medically assisted death has become the "new normal" for a death with dignity and a "good death," there is an urgent need to educate Catholics that physician-performed euthanasia and medically assisted suicide are the rejection of the Paschal Mystery, the suffering, death, and resurrection of Jesus Christ (Rolheiser, 2015). Jesus's suffering is real, life giving, and redemptive. We do not seek suffering; we have a duty to relieve it where possible but believe that through our pain and suffering, we can share in the redemptive work of Christ.

Canadian Catholics have learned the need to educate and reclaim a "good death" for our time, which is secular and which believes in the power of science and technology to save. Christians envisioned the good death of Saint Joseph, a "righteous man" who lived in fidelity to God's call, cared for by his beloved Mary and Jesus, in a scene of both sadness and deep trust in the faithfulness of God. In medieval times, when death came suddenly to most, Christians prepared for a good death through the *ars moriendi* (O'Conner, 1966). This "art of dying" depended upon two cultural features: shared faith in the life, salvific suffering, death, and resurrection of Jesus as the ultimate sign of God's love for us and the centrality of families and community in care for the sick and dying. Our pluralist and secular culture is very different: a religious worldview is no longer shared; healthcare is professionalized; individual rights, choice, and control are primary values; and there is widespread belief in technology to cure all our ills.

These simpler times seem far from our experience of seemingly death-defying medical advances. However, the features patients and families have described of a good death today include pain and symptom management; respectful communication; and opportunities to achieve their personal and spiritual "bucket list" of farewells, reconciliation, and giving and receiving expressions of love, gratitude, and forgiveness (Steinhauser et al., 2000). Palliative care, provided in hospices, hospitals, homes, and communities, was developed to support the dying, where death was considered a failure, and technology dominated care (Byock, 2013). As palliative care specialists affirm in other chapters in this book, its original goals promised to neither hasten nor prolong dying. Catholics in Canada have learned the importance of advocacy for hospice and palliative care as an alternative to medically assisted death. In the Canadian context, we have learned that once medically assisted death was legalized, patient expressions of interest in "ending it" resulted in a clinical response that moved to assessment of eligibility for the procedure rather than a reassessment of the patient's care and management, including attention to spiritual issues. Crucially important is the recognition that requests for medically assisted death may come with no or very late palliative care consultation (Seller, Bouthillier, & Fraser, 2018).

Palliative care itself is threatened because medically assisted death has been legalized in Canada before delivery of the government promise to ensure access to effective hospice and palliative care as a right of all Canadian residents. Money needed to support research into difficult end-of-life care and to develop standards of care for urban and rural situations is threatened by economic benefits of medically assisted death. This is of particular importance in single-payer and tax-supported health systems. More generally, Sulmasy has reflected on healthcare justice, emphasizing the values of human dignity, compassion, solidarity, and the common good. He identifies humans as naturally social, yielding a principle of solidarity; finite, requiring dying and death to be taken seriously; and "hav[ing] a radically equal intrinsic worth or dignity that commands the respect of others, independent of our preferences" (2003).

Other authors in this book review crucially important work on "dignity-preserving care," including Canadian Dr. Harvey Chochinov's pioneer research, which has focused on understanding what is meant by loss of dignity and which attitudes and practices foster dignity or erode it in serious and terminal illness (2012). All these issues need to be taken into account to restore a sense of dignity and worth in a patient's final days. Life may have been lived without dignity, but dying can be truly dignified.

Canadians have also learned the need to resist the failure of promised conscience protection for practitioners who object to medically assisted death. Conscience is not about competing rights but developing moral insight and courage, without which protection of those most vulnerable to medically assisted death is compromised.

Prophetic resistance demands prophetic witness. We must accept that

> An evangelizing community . . . has an endless desire to show mercy, the fruit of its own experience of the power of the Father's infinite mercy. . . . An evangelizing community gets involved by word and deed in people's lives; it bridges distances, it is willing to abase itself if necessary and it embraces human life, touching the suffering flesh of Christ in others. An evangelizing community is also supportive, standing by people at every step of the way, no matter how difficult or lengthy this may prove to be.
>
> *(Apostolic Exhortation,* 2013)

Prophetic witness is needed in direct care for and accompaniment of the sick, suffering, and vulnerable as part of our baptismal call. Canadians have learned we must be active and vigilant in protection of the vulnerable from medically assisted death.

Discussion Questions

1. How does the author define dignity?
2. What qualifies as death with dignity?

References

Apostolic Exhortation: Evangelii Gaudium. (2013). No. 24. www.zenit.org.

Beyleveld, D., & Brownsword, R. (2001). *Human Dignity in Bioethics and Biolaw.* Oxford: Oxford University Press.

Brown, K. (2011). "Vulnerability": Handle with care. *Ethics and Social Welfare* 5(3), 313–321.

Brown, R. E. (1994). *The Death of the Messiah: From Gethsemane to the Grave: A Commentary on the Passion in the Four Gospels,* 2 Vols. New York: Doubleday.

Bruggemann, W. (2001). *The Prophetic Imagination,* 2nd ed. Minneapolis, MN: Fortress Press.

Byers, P. (2016). Dependence and a Kantian conception of dignity as a value. *Theoretical Medicine and Bioethics* 37(1), 61–69.

Byock, I. (2013). *The Best Care Possible.* New York: Avery.

Carter v. Canada (Attorney General). (2015). SCC 5, 1 SCR 331, 35591.

Carter, S. L. (1993). *The Culture of Disbelief: How American Law and Politics Trivialize Religious Devotion.* New York: Doubleday.

Cassell, E. J. (1991). *The Nature of Suffering and the Goals of Medicine.* Oxford: Oxford University Press.

Catechism of the Catholic Church. (n.d.). No. 27. www.vatican.va/archive/ENG0015/_ INDEX.HTM.

Chochinov, H. M. (2012). *Dignity Therapy: Final Words for Final Days.* New York: Oxford University Press.

Dignitas Personae. (2008). No 7–8. www.zenit.org.

Dresser, R. (2009). Human dignity and the seriously ill patient. In E. D. Pellegrino, A. Schulman, & T. W. Merrill (Eds.), *Human Dignity and Bioethics,* 505–512. Notre Dame, IN: University of Notre Dame Press.

Emanuel, E. J., Fairclough, D. L., & Emanuel, L. L. (2000). Attitudes and desires related to euthanasia and physician assisted suicide among terminally ill patients and their caregivers. *JAMA – Journal of the American Medical Association* 284(19), 2460–2468.

Evangelium Vitae. (1995). No. 3. www.zenit.org.

Fukuyama, F. (2002). *Our Posthuman Future: Consequences of the Biotechnology Revolution.* New York: Farrar, Straus & Giroux.

Ganzini, L., Gay, E. R., & Dobscha. S. K. (2008). Why Oregon patients request assisted death: Family members views. *Journal of General Internal Medicine* 23(2), 154–157.

Gawande, A. (2014). *Being Mortal: Medicine and What Matters in the End.* Toronto, ON: Doubleday Canada.

Gerlenter, D. (2009). The irreducibly religious character of human dignity. In E. D. Pellegrino, A. Schulman, & T. W. Merrill (Eds.), *Human Dignity and Bioethics,* 387–405. Notre Dame, IN: University of Notre Dame Press.

Hunter, K. M. (1993). *Doctors' Stories: The Narrative Structure of Medical Knowledge.* Princeton, NJ: Princeton University Press.

Kass, L. R. (2002). *Life, Liberty and the Defense of Dignity: The Challenge for Bioethics*. San Francisco, CA: Encounter Books.

Kenny, N. (2017). *Rediscovering the Art of Dying: How Jesus' Experience and Our Stories Reveal a New Vision of Compassionate Care*. Toronto, ON: Novalis.

Kleinman, A. (1988). *The Illness Narratives: Suffering, Healing and the Human Condition*. New York: Basic Books Harper Collins.

Lazenby, M., McCorkindale, R., & Sulmasy, D. P. (Eds.). (2014). *Safe Passage: A Global Spiritual Sourcebook for Care at the End of Life*. Oxford: Oxford University Press.

Lotz, M. (2016). Vulnerability and resilience: A critical nexus. *Theoretical Medicine and Bioethics* 37(1), 45–59.

Mackenie, C., Rogers, W., & Dodds, S. (Eds.). (2013). *Vulnerability: New Essays in Ethics and Feminist Philosophy*. Oxford: Oxford University Press.

Macklin, R. (2003). Dignity is a useless concept. *British Medical Journal* 327(7429), 1419–1420.

Martin, J. (2014). *Jesus: A Pilgrimage*. New York: Harper Collins.

Matthews, S., & Tobin, B. (2016). Human vulnerability in medical contexts. *Theoretical Medicine and Bioethics* 37(1), 1–7.

Meilander, G. (2007, Summer). Human dignity and public bioethics. *New Atlantis* 33–52. www.thenewatlantis.com/publications/human-dignity-and-public-bioethics.

O'Conner, M. C. (1966). *The Art of Dying Well: The Development of the Ars Moriendi*. New York: AMS Press.

Pellegrino, E. D., Schulman, A., & Merrill, T. W. (Eds.). (2009). *Human Dignity and Bioethics*. Notre Dame, IN: University of Notre Dame Press.

Pellegrino, E. D., & Thomasma, D. C. (1988). *For the Patient's Good: The Restoration of Beneficence in Health Care*. New York: Oxford University Press.

Rolheiser, R. (2015). *The Passion and the Cross*. Toronto, ON: Novalis.

Salvifici Doloris. (1984). Sec. 5. www.zenit.org.

Schulman, A. (2009). Bioethics and the question of human dignity. In E. D. Pellegrino, A. Schulman, & T. W. Merrill (Eds.), *Human Dignity and Bioethics*, 3–18. Notre Dame, IN: University of Notre Dame Press.

Seller, L., Bouthillier, M. E., & Fraser, V. (2018). Situating requests for medical aid in dying within the broader context of end of life care: Ethical considerations. *Journal of Medical Ethics* 45(2), 106–111.

Steinhauser, K. E., Christakis, N. A., Clipp, E. C., McNeilly, M., McIntryre, L., & Tulsky, J. A. (2000). Factors considered important at the end of life by patients, family, physicians, and other care providers. *JAMA – Journal of the American Medical Association* 284(19), 2476–2482.

Sulmasy, D. P. (2002). Death, dignity and the theory of value. *Ethical Perspectives* 9(2–3), 103–118.

Sulmasy, D. P. (2003). Health care justice and hospice care. *Hastings Center Report* 33(2), S14–5 (special supplement).

United Nations General Assembly. (1948, December 10). *Universal Declaration of Human Rights*. www.un.org/en/universal-declaration-human-rights/.

Chapter 14

Health Policy Considerations for Spiritual Care in the United States

Howard K. Koh and Eric Coles

A growing body of evidence links spirituality (however it is defined) with improved health outcomes. On the other hand, burnout, often linked with a loss of spirituality, affects many caregivers, who may lack the time, training, and confidence to deal with their patients' spiritual difficulties as well as their own. Current efforts by the Veterans Administration, the Faith and Opportunity Initiative, and the Affordable Care Act show promise in how to increase spirituality in care to the benefit of all.

As far back as 350 BCE, Aristotle put forward his philosophy that the soul is the full actualization of a person, incorporating the body, the purpose, and ultimately the sum of total operations of being human (Aristotle, 2012). In 1946, the World Health Organization (WHO) defined health as "a state of complete physical, mental and social well-being and not merely the absence of disease or infirmity." That same year, the WHO noted that "the enjoyment of the highest attainable standard of health is one of the fundamental rights of every human being" (World Health Organization, 1946).

These profound perspectives help us view the status of health in the United States today. The United States has the most expensive healthcare system in the world, without the health outcomes to match (Squires, 2015). Suboptimal outcomes and fragmented care, covered by largely fee-for-service insurance, have prompted national debate on better ways to improve the health of the nation. President Barack Obama signed the Affordable Care Act (ACA) into law on March 23, 2010. Although its passage has led to 20 million more Americans covered by health insurance, debate continues about how best to create a system that can provide high-quality, value-based, person-centered care.

Moving toward this goal should involve policies that promote complete well-being, not merely the absence of disease, to recognize the total operations of being human. Returning to a time that respects the spiritual dimensions of complete well-being could help more people reach their "highest attainable standard of health" (World Health Organization, 1946).

Spirituality and Spiritual Care

An international consensus conference has defined spirituality as "a dynamic intrinsic aspect of humanity through which persons seek ultimate meaning, purpose and transcendence." In 2017, VanderWeele, Balboni, and I (Koh) wrote an article in the *Journal of the American Medical Association* to revisit and reaffirm some critical themes at the intersection between health and spirituality (VanderWeele, Balboni, & Koh, 2017).

Studies note that the vast majority of patients find spirituality important in their lives (Astrow, Kwok, Sharma, Fromer, & Sulmasy, 2018). People can discover ultimate meaning and purpose through their interactions with family, in the community, while convening with nature, or at work. A more formal way involves religion. In the United States, a nation of 330 million people, 77 percent indicate a religious affiliation; this population is about 46 percent Protestant, 21 percent Catholic, 2 percent Jewish, and about 1 percent both Muslim and Hindu. Moreover, about a third attend religious services weekly (Lipka, 2015).

Recognizing a person's spirituality involves acknowledging religious and other considerations related to what a person considers to be of ultimate meaning, purpose, and transcendence. Respecting human dignity – "an internal state of peace that comes with the recognition and acceptance of the value and vulnerability of all living things" – in this way involves accepting the identity of others, treating people fairly and equally, empowering others, and holding oneself accountable for transgressions (Hicks, 2011). But busy clinicians may find honoring dignity most challenging in hectic practices that easily lead to dehumanization. The late Reverend William Sloane Coffin once warned that physicians shouldn't view a patient as "an uninteresting appendage to an interesting disease" (Jarvis & Johnson, 2013).

A growing body of evidence links spirituality (defined in various ways) with improved health outcomes. For example, one study of over 74,000 participants from the Nurses Health Study (1992–2012) found that regular religious service attendance was associated with a 20–35 percent reduction in all-cause mortality, as well as risk reductions for depression and suicide of 30 percent and 84 percent, respectively (VanderWeele, 2017). Also, a meta-analysis of ten prospective studies involving about 136,000 participants found that having a sense of purpose in life is associated with an adjusted reduced risk for all-cause mortality and cardiovascular events (0.83) (Cohen, Bavishi, & Rozanski, 2016). As a recent systematic review of specific spiritual care interventions noted only small benefits for patients; however, more research is needed (Kruizinga et al., 2016).

Studies also note that illness can be a time of spiritual distress, a theme too often ignored by medical providers. In a study of over 700 racially, ethnically, and religiously diverse participants, nearly eight in ten reported spiritual needs;

those with higher burdens reported less satisfaction with the care they received (Astrow et al., 2018). Another study found that spiritual distress leads to more psychological distress during difficult life events (Trevino, Pargament, Krause, Ironson, & Hill, 2017).

Spiritual distress is not necessarily restricted to patients. Issues of burnout currently affect physicians and, indeed, all types of caregivers. One survey indicated that 60 percent of physicians were considering leaving practice for a variety of reasons (Lucian Leape Institute, 2013). Another article quotes one doctor as saying "at the highest level, we are disconnected from our purpose and have lost touch with the things that give joy and meaning to our work" (Wright & Katz, 2018).

Creating guidelines for spiritual care in practice and broader policy for populations will require addressing fundamental issues about data, evidence, feasibility, workforce, training, and reimbursement. For example, chaplains can provide valuable spiritual care services, and almost all major hospitals now have hospital chaplain services. However, chaplain profiles can vary widely, and they usually cannot bill or be specifically reimbursed for services; an upcoming study from the National Institutes of Health will evaluate hospital chaplaincy in palliative care for the first time (Healthcare Chaplaincy Network, 2016).

Meanwhile, physicians and other medical providers could serve as valuable healers for spiritual distress, but they report that they lack the time, training, and confidence to do so. As the field still remains embryonic, critical research can explore what constitutes spiritual care, how it can be implemented, for whom and by whom, and when.

The Clinical Setting

A recent review of the state of the science of spiritual care research recommends developing two clinical areas: 1) spiritual screening and obtaining spiritual history, which can be brief and offered by a clinical provider, and 2) if needed, a deeper spiritual assessment through referral to a specialist who is a certified spiritual care professional (Steinhauser et al., 2017).

Regarding the first phase, effective tools for spiritual screening could include a number of options. One study recommends communication that addresses eight domains, including understanding goals, fears, and worries; an opening question to patients could be, "What are your biggest fears and worries about the future with your health?" (Bernacki & Block, 2014). Puchalski and colleagues have led development of a spiritual history intake tool that asks about faith and belief as part of care (Puchalski, 2013). The authors created a guide for conversation for spiritual assessment known as FICA, which represents faith, importance, community, and address. Recommended questions are offered for each phase, such as "How would you like me as your provider to address spirituality in your healthcare?"

Information regarding screening and evaluation of patients' spiritual needs can now be integrated into electronic health records (EHRs) (National Association of Catholic Chaplains, 2019). Hospital chaplains have differing levels of access to, and familiarity with, EHRs. And without a standard protocol, key questions remain about how best to assess and document spiritual needs in times of illness (Tartaglia, Dodd-McCue, Ford, Demm, & Hassell, 2016).

With respect to spiritual challenges for clinicians, a group of CEOs of leading healthcare organizations has committed to begin by measuring physician well-being (Noseworthy, Madara, Cosgrove, Edgeworth, & Ellison, 2017). And from an organizational perspective, some researchers suggest that "meaning" join previously noted overarching goals of "better health, better care, and lower costs" as part of a new "quadruple aim" (Bodenheimer & Sinsky, 2014).

Hospice and Palliative Care

The first hospice in the United States was founded in the 1970s by Florence Wald and colleagues, including Reverend Edward Dobihal, chaplain of Yale-New Haven Hospital. Currently in the United States, there are 4000 hospices, known as a place of shelter and restful reality for travelers on a long journey. Research has demonstrated that hospice care for cancer patients in the last year of life can lower hospitalization rates, intensive care unit admissions, invasive procedures, and costs (Emanuel et al., 2002). In 1982, the Medicare Hospice Benefit was established and then updated in 1986. The benefit, for those with fewer than six months to live, covers costs of noncurative care. Its overall benefit of about $200 a day does not specifically address spiritual care needs (National Hospice and Palliative Care Organization, 2016).

As noted by the WHO, palliative care improves quality of life for patients and families and relieves suffering from spiritual pain, in addition to treating physical and psychosocial pain. Recent studies show that about 67 percent of US hospitals now offer palliative care services (Dumanovsky et al., 2015). A landmark 2015 Institute of Medicine (IOM) report, *Dying in America*, suggests that the core components of end-of-life care include frequent assessment of patient's spiritual well-being, which includes attention to patients' spiritual and religious needs (Institute of Medicine, 2014).

Such attention to spirituality in end-of-life care has bearing on many issues, ranging from medical interventions and healthcare costs to basic considerations about human dignity. One study, using support from religious communities as a proxy for spirituality, found that terminally ill patients with high religious community support accessed hospice care less and aggressive medical interventions more than patients without support (Phelps et al., 2009). Other studies found that religiousness, a proxy for spirituality, is associated with less advanced-care planning and more aggressive medical interventions in terminally ill adults (Balboni et al., 2007). These results have major implications for healthcare costs, especially since approximately a third of Medicare spending involves chronically ill people in their last two years of life (Griffin, 2016).

Also, in the end-of-life setting, healthcare providers may not necessarily be following patient preferences. One survey of seriously ill patients found that of patients who requested to die at home, a majority of them actually died in a hospital (Dartmouth Atlas Project, 2019). More explicit attention to desired care, especially when the patient is unable to speak for himself/herself, is critical to honoring dignity. Advanced directives, usually in the form of living wills or healthcare powers of attorney, have only been completed by about one in three Americans (Yadav et al., 2017).

In 2016, Medicare announced that its physician fee schedule would include new, separate billing codes for advanced-care planning, representing a critical step forward for policy. Early studies have found, however, only a modest, if any, uptake in physicians billing for such conversations (Tsai & Taylor, 2018). Obstacles to large-scale change included low visibility, lengthy documentation, and professional norms.

The IOM report also offers five key recommendations for spiritual care as part of palliative care. One recommendation, ensuring insurance coverage of comprehensive care at the end of life, specifically addresses spiritual and religious needs. The other four (related to quality clinician–patient communication, professional education, certification and licensure, and payment systems) could be expanded in the future to explicitly address needed spiritual care (Institute of Medicine, 2014).

The United States Department of Veterans Affairs Health System

The Department of Veterans Affairs (VA), the largest US integrated health system, with 170 medical centers and over 1000 outpatient sites, has prioritized spiritual and pastoral care. From 2002 to 2017, the VA witnessed substantial growth in its hospice and palliative care services. Interdisciplinary palliative care teams offer support in every VA facility, and the system features close to 100 dedicated inpatient hospice units (Parker, 2019). A chaplain, part of the palliative care team addressing psychological, emotional, social, and spiritual needs, represents a key emphasis of the VA health culture. Spiritual care in the VA also extends to patient populations with suicide risk and posttraumatic stress disorder.

The VA's palliative care program uses the National Bereaved Family Survey as part of its evaluation. The survey of about 9000 individuals shows that about 90 percent of families desire spiritual support; the great majority receive it. The survey includes a question regarding how well the spiritual needs of the patient were met (US Department of Veteran Affairs, 2018). Such evaluation contributes to emerging quality measures for palliative care (Dy et al., 2015).

The 2018 Creating High-Quality Results and Outcomes Necessary to Improve Chronic (CHRONIC) Care Act (Chernof & McClellan, 2018) brings recent attention to Medicare payment for some nonmedical services (e.g., food, transportation) and expands reimbursement for Independence at Home programs. Specifically, Medicare Advantage plans can now cover some non-medical costs, allowing more consideration for other determinants of well-being, such as spiritual care.

The CHRONIC Act changes Medicare Advantage supplemental benefit coverage from care that is "primarily designed to prevent, cure or diminish an illness or injury" to services that aid "a reasonable expectation of improving or maintaining the health or overall function of the chronically ill enrollee and may not be limited to being primarily health-related benefits" (Willink & DuGoff, 2018). And regarding to spiritual care, the bill includes language that "interdisciplinary care teams may include a chaplain, minister or other clergy" (Hatch, 2017). The act marks an important step in the transition to paying for the value of care, but how such developments can affect spiritual care remains to be seen.

Other future avenues to address spiritual care integration could potentially involve demonstration projects sponsored by the Center for Medicare and Medicaid Innovation (CMMI). The ACA created the CMMI to test new alternative payment models as an option for traditional fee-for-service. Such models now include accountable care organizations and accountable health communities; the latter addresses health-related model social needs in providing care to defined populations (Alley, Asomugha, Conway, & Sanghavi, 2016). Incorporating spiritual care into demonstration projects to determine impact on quality and costs could be an avenue for future applied research.

Another potential venue involves the White House Faith and Opportunity Initiative, formerly the Office of Faith-Based and Neighborhood Partnerships established by the Bush administration in 2001 and extended through the Obama administration up to the present day (White House, 2018). Previously, this office had encouraged federal agencies to collaborate with faith-based organizations, provided that inherently religious activities (e.g., prayer, worship) are not funded by the government and that other conditions outlined in the First Amendment's Establishment Clause are not violated. This bipartisan effort has led to partnerships for a wide range of health promotion and social service activities (Koh & Coles, 2019). In a time where communities are wrestling with the opioid crisis, substance use disorders, cirrhosis, self-harm, and other so-called "diseases of despair," addressing the spiritual underpinnings of such conditions could represent a potential avenue of work (Moreau, 2018).

Conclusion

A future vision of spiritual care could arise by addressing basic questions about what, why, how, who and for whom, when, and why. For example, more research can address issues of patient-centered communication and care to identify spiritual needs and distress. Doing so could enhance dimensions of quality in care and value for the patient while cultivating dignity for patients and clinicians alike. A generalist-specialist model, team-based and coordinated, could potentially bring together medical and spiritual care providers to offer better person-centered services. Such efforts, potentially valuable for anyone, could be especially critical for end-of-life situations.

Moving toward such a vision will require much more dialogue, consensus, research, funding, and national commitment. Advancing policies to move the conversation forward can be one way to promote complete well-being for patients and populations in the future.

Discussion Questions

1. What is the significance of palliative care in public health ethics?
2. How does public health influence spirituality in palliative care?

References

Alley, D. E., Asomugha, C. N., Conway, P. H., & Sanghavi, D. M. (2016). Accountable health communities – Addressing social needs through Medicare and Medicaid. *New England Journal of Medicine* 374(1), 8–11. https://doi.org/10.1056/NEJM p1512532.

Aristotle. (2012). *De Anima: On the Soul*. Translated by Mark Shiffman. Amazon Digital Services. Originally published c. 350 BCE.

Astrow, A. B., Kwok, G., Sharma, R. K., Fromer, N., & Sulmasy, D. P. (2018). Spiritual needs and perception of quality of care and satisfaction with care in hematology/medical oncology patients: A multicultural assessment. *Journal of Pain and Symptom Management* 55(1), 56–64.

Balboni, T. A., Vanderwerker, L. C., Block, S. D., Paulk, M. E., Lathan, C. S., Peteet, J. R., & Prigerson, H. G. (2007). Religiousness and spiritual support among advanced cancer patients and associations with end-of-life treatment preferences and quality of life. *Journal of Clinical Oncology* 25(5), 555.

Bernacki, R. E., & Block, S. D. (2014). Communication about serious illness care goals: A review and synthesis of best practices. *JAMA Internal Medicine* 174(12), 1994–2003.

Bodenheimer, T., & Sinsky, C. (2014). From triple to quadruple aim: Care of the patient requires care of the provider. *Annals of Family Medicine* 12(6), 573–576. https://doi.org/10.1370/afm.1713.

Chernof, B., & McClellan, M. B. (2018, August 10). Form follows funding: Opportunities for advancing outcomes for complex care patients using alternative payment methods. *Health Affairs*. www.healthaffairs.org/do/10.1377/hblog20180803.928422/full/.

Cohen, R., Bavishi, C., & Rozanski, A. (2016). Purpose in life and its relationship to all-cause mortality and cardiovascular events: A meta-analysis. *Psychosomatic Medicine* 78(2), 122. https://doi.org/10.1097/PSY.0000000000000274.

Dartmouth Atlas Project. (2019). End of life care. *Dartmouth Atlas of Health Care* (blog). www.dartmouthatlas.org/interactive-apps/end-of-life-care/.

Dumanovsky, T., Augustin, R., Rogers, M., Lettang, K., Meier, D. E., & Morrison, R. S. (2015). The growth of palliative care in U.S. hospitals: A status report. *Journal of Palliative Medicine* 19(1), 8–15. https://doi.org/10.1089/jpm.2015.0351.

Dy, S. M., Kiley, K. B., Ast, K., Lupu, D., Norton, S. A., McMillan, S. C., . . . Casarett, D. J. (2015). Measuring what matters: Top-ranked quality indicators for hospice and palliative care from the American Academy of Hospice and Palliative Medicine and Hospice and Palliative Nurses Association. *Journal of Pain and Symptom Management* 49(4), 773–781. https://doi.org/10.1016/j.jpainsymman.2015.01.012.

Emanuel, E. J., Ash, A., Yu, W., Gazelle, G., Levinsky, N. G., Saynina, O., . . . Moskowitz, M. (2002). Managed care, hospice use, site of death, and medical expenditures in the last year of life. *Archives of Internal Medicine* 162(15), 1722–1728.

Griffin, S. (2016, July 14). Medicare spending at the end of life: A snapshot of beneficiaries who died in 2014 and the cost of their care. *Henry J. Kaiser Family Foundation* (blog). www.kff.org/medicare/issue-brief/medicare-spending-at-the-end-of-life/.

Hatch, O. G. (2017, September 29). S.870–115th Congress (2017–2018): Creating High-Quality Results and Outcomes Necessary to Improve Chronic (CHRONIC) Care Act of 2017. Webpage. www.congress.gov/bill/115th-congress/senate-bill/870.

Healthcare Chaplaincy Network. (2016, December). National Institutes of Health funds study of spiritual care in palliative care. *Press Release*. www.healthcarechaplaincy.org/docs/research/dignity_therapy_project_announcement_12_16.pdf.

Hicks, D. (2011). *Dignity: The Essential Role It Plays in Resolving Conflict*. New Haven, CT: Yale University Press.

Institute of Medicine. (2014). *Dying in America: Improving Quality and Honoring Individual Preferences Near the End of Life*. Washington, DC: National Academies Press.

Jarvis, C. A., & Johnson, E. (2013). *Feasting on the Gospels – Matthew: A Feasting on the Word Commentary*, vol. 1. Louisville, KY: Westminster John Knox Press.

Koh, H. K., & Coles, E. (2019). Body and soul: Health collaborations with faith-based organizations. *American Journal of Public Health* 109(3), 369–370.

Kruizinga, R., Hartog, I. D., Jacobs, M., Daams, J. G., Scherer-Rath, M., Schilderman, J. B. A. M., . . . Van Laarhoven, H. W. M. (2016). The effect of spiritual interventions addressing existential themes using a narrative approach on quality of life of cancer patients: A systematic review and meta-analysis. *Psycho-Oncology* 25(3), 253–265. https://doi.org/10.1002/pon.3910.

Lipka, M. (2015, May 12). 5 key findings about the changing U.S. religious landscape. *Pew Research Center* (blog). www.pewresearch.org/fact-tank/2015/05/12/5-key-findings-u-s-religious-landscape/.

Lucian Leape Institute. (2013). Institute for healthcare improvement: Through the eyes of the workforce: Creating joy, meaning, and safer health care. www.ihi.org:80/resources/Pages/Publications/Through-the-Eyes-of-the-Workforce-Creating-Joy-Meaning-and-Safer-Health-Care.aspx.

Moreau, J. (2018, May 7). Civil rights groups wary of Trump's latest faith-based initiative. *NBC News*. www.nbcnews.com/feature/nbc-out/civil-rights-groups-wary-trump-s-latest-faith-based-initiative-n872031.

National Association of Catholic Chaplains. (2019). EMR spiritual assessments. *National Association of Catholic Chaplains* (blog). www.nacc.org/resources/chaplaincy-care-resources/spiritual-assessments-and-emr/emr-spiritual-assessments-no-epic-content/.

National Hospice and Palliative Care Organization. (2016). *History of Hospice Care*. National Hospice and Palliative Care Organization. www.nhpco.org/history-hospice-care.

Noseworthy, J., Madara, J., Cosgrove, D., Edgeworth, M., & Ellison, E. (2017, March 28). Physician burnout is a public health crisis: A message to our fellow health care CEOs. *Health Affairs Blog*. www.healthaffairs.org/do/10.1377/hblog20170328.059397/full/.

Parker, J. (2019, April 9). VA to expand hospice, palliative care for veterans. *Hospice News*. https://hospicenews.com/2019/04/09/va-to-expand-hospice-palliative-care-for-veterans/.

Phelps, A. C., Maciejewski, P. K., Nilsson, M., Balboni, T. A., Wright, A. A., Paulk, M. E., . . . Block, S. D. (2009). Religious coping and use of intensive life-prolonging care near death in patients with advanced cancer. *JAMA – Journal of the American Medical Association* 301(11), 1140–1147.

Puchalski, C. M. (2013). The FICA spiritual history tool #274. *Journal of Palliative Medicine* 17(1), 105–106. https://doi.org/10.1089/jpm.2013.9458.

Squires, D. (2015). Spending, use of services, prices, and health in 13 countries. *Commonwealth Fund*. www.commonwealthfund.org/publications/issue-briefs/2015/oct/us-health-care-global-perspective.

Steinhauser, K. E., Fitchett, G., Handzo, G. F., Johnson, K. S., Koenig, H. G., Pargament, K. I., . . . Balboni, T. A. (2017). State of the science of spirituality and palliative care research, part I: Definitions, measurement, and outcomes. *Journal of Pain and Symptom Management* 54(3), 428–440.

Tartaglia, A., Dodd-McCue, D., Ford, T., Demm, C., & Hassell, A. (2016). Chaplain documentation and the electronic medical record: A survey of ACPE residency programs. *Journal of Health Care Chaplaincy* 22(2), 41–53. https://doi.org/10.1080/08854726.2015.1071544.

Trevino, K. M., Pargament, K. I., Krause, N., Ironson, G., & Hill, P. (2017). Stressful events and religious/spiritual struggle: Moderating effects of the general orienting system. *Psychology of Religion and Spirituality*. http://dx.doi.org/10.1037/rel0000149.

Tsai, G., & Taylor, D. H. (2018). Advance care planning in Medicare: An early look at the impact of new reimbursement on billing and clinical practice. *BMJ Supportive & Palliative Care* 8(1), 49–52.

US Department of Veteran Affairs. (2018). *The Bereaved Family Survey – Inpatient – Center for Health Equity Research and Promotion*. General Information. www.cherp.research.va.gov/PROMISE/The_PROMISE_Survey.asp.

VanderWeele, T. J. (2017). Religion and health: A synthesis. In M. J. Balboni & J. R. Peteet (Eds.), *Spirituality and Religion within the Culture of Medicine: From Evidence to Practice*, 357–402. Oxford: Oxford University Press.

VanderWeele, T. J., Balboni, T. A., & Koh, H. K. (2017). Health and Spirituality. *JAMA – Journal of the American Medical Association* 318(6), 519–520.

White House. (2018, May 3). *Executive Order on the Establishment of a White House Faith and Opportunity Initiative*. White House. www.whitehouse.gov/presidential-actions/executive-order-establishment-white-house-faith-opportunity-initiative/.

Willink, A., & DuGoff, E. H. (2018). Integrating medical and nonmedical services: The promise and pitfalls of the CHRONIC Care Act. *New England Journal of Medicine* 378(23), 2153–2155. https://doi.org/10.1056/NEJMp1803292.

World Health Organization. (1946). *Constitution of WHO: Principles*. WHO. www. who.int/about/mission/en/.

Wright, A. A., & Katz, I. T. (2018, March 30). Beyond burnout: Redesigning care to restore meaning and sanity. *NEJM Catalyst*. www.nejm.org/doi/full/10.1056/ NEJMp1716845.

Yadav, K. N., Gabler, N. B., Cooney, E., Kent, S., Kim, J., Herbst, N., . . . Courtright, K. R. 2017. Approximately one in three US adults completes any type of advance directive for end-of-life care. *Health Affairs* 36(7), 1244–1251. https://doi.org/10.1377/ hlthaff.2017.0175.

Chapter 15

Pediatrics and Aging

Palliative Care

Franca Benini and Ferdinando Cancelli

Care requirements for pediatric patients are different from those of adult and/or the elderly. For one thing, care must be provided through several stages, from infant to teenager, with all the concomitant developmental issues. Because of the limited number of patients, medical care can be spread over a vast geographic area. The effects on family, who bear social and financial burdens, are tremendous. A pediatric palliative care network that brings together children, families, and caregivers would help solve many of these problems.

At the other end of the spectrum, there are growing numbers of elderly patients in need of palliative care, especially those with chronic and degenerative conditions. One-quarter of people aged 85 years and older have dementia, which can last from 2 to 15 years, placing a tremendous financial and caregiving burden on family members. Side effects of medications are complicated by the number and severity of other chronic conditions. Within geriatric treatment, care can be subdivided into slow, gradual, and rapid decline, each of which has specific concerns for an increasingly frail person.

Pediatric Palliative Care

Franca Benini

In recent years, there have been gradual but continuous transformations in care needs in pediatric medicine: a new type of patient, different settings, and diverse "healthcare" goals. One of these "innovations" is the need for palliative care (PC) in the child population.

The developed world has seen an increase in the prevalence of incurable disease and disability. Medical and technological advances have reduced infant and child mortality rates and, at the same time, have improved the survival of children with severe and potentially lethal pathologies.

These are babies, children, and young people affected by a wide range of serious medical conditions for which no curative treatment options are available. Frequently they live with multiple organ failure together with cognitive and/or neurodegenerative problems and, often, are technologically dependent on medical "devices" to compensate for the loss of a vital bodily function and substantial and ongoing nursing care to avert death or further disability.

These babies, children, and young adults have unique and complex needs that require combined multidisciplinary and inter-institutional care that comes under the umbrella of pediatric palliative care (PPC), where the focus is on safeguarding the best "quality of life" possible for the child and family (Goldman, Hain, & Liben, 2012; Wolfe, Jones, Kreicbergs, & Jankovic, 2018; Field & Behrman, 2003; Friedrichsdorf & Bruera, 2018).

Definitions

The World Health Organization (WHO) defines children's palliative care as "The active total care of the child's body, mind and spirit, and also involves providing support to the family." The objective is the best quality of life possible for the child and family and, in the vast majority of cases, the family home represents the best setting for care delivery.

PPC is not just care of the dying, which refers to care during the last phases of a terminal illness and into bereavement, but foresees support from early in the progression of a potentially fatal illness. It begins at diagnosis; it does not preclude treatment aimed at a cure or prolonging life and should continue throughout the course of the illness. PPC embraces all the physical, emotional, social, and spiritual elements that are linked to serious illness and the death of a child.

To be effective, PPC must be provided by an experienced interdisciplinary and multispecialist team capable of providing multifaceted care solutions delivered across a selection of healthcare settings (hospital, hospice, home) (Himelstein, Hilden, Boldt, & Weissman, 2004; European Association of Palliative Care, 2007).

The Particularity of Pediatric Palliative Care

PPC differs in many ways from palliative care for adults, as it must be tailored to the child's biological, psycho-relational, clinical, social, ethical, and spiritual needs throughout their development (newborn, child, or adolescent) and must address a multitude of unique and individual needs that condition care choices and treatments (Himelstein et al., 2004; European Association of Palliative Care, 2007).

Some of the aspects that distinguish children's palliative care are the following.

The uniqueness and complexity of interventions: Children are individuals in continuous evolution (from neonates to young adults). They continually develop at physical, cognitive, emotional, social, and spiritual levels, which influences all aspects of their care – including pharmacological treatment, communication, and their dependency on others. Consequently, care programs must be flexible and tailored to individual needs; each intervention and care choice needs to be adapted to the biological, cognitive, psycho-relational, social, ethical, and spiritual peculiarities of the specific development phase in order to respond appropriately to the diverse types and quantities of needs and to address individual issues.

The types of conditions and duration of care: The spectrum of conditions eligible for PPC are multiple and wide ranging (neuromuscular, neurode-generative, cancer, metabolic disorders, chromosomal abnormalities, cardiovascular anomalies, respiratory and infectious diseases, complications of prematurity, and trauma), which means that the duration of care is immensely variable and difficult to predict (sometimes many years). The treatments required are multifaceted and specific to a childhood condition; many of these illnesses are exclusive to the pediatric age since the children affected rarely reach adulthood, where palliative care is provided predominantly for patients with cancer.

The role of the family: The parents represent their children in all the choices that concern them; they are at the center of all communication and, if the child is living at home, the majority of care provision is delegated to them. While coming to terms and coping with the tragedy of their child's incurable illness, they must become a reference point for their children: the family must make arrangements for the child's care, social needs, and fulfillment of their wishes. The family plays a decisive role in creating a network of caregivers, friends, and family that has the potential to greatly impact the quality of life and death of their child.

Ethical and legal implications: For adult patients, from the ethical, scientific, legislative, deontological, and operational points of view, it has long since been recognized and established that, except in few exceptional cases, all care/treatment choices must be discussed, planned, and agreed upon with the patient. However, when the patient is a child, the criticalities and limitations faced in this matter are undeniably complex and manifold (mainly directly linked to the age and clinical condition of the child patient). Some concepts and circumstances such as quality of life, best interests, self-termination, autonomy, and limits in the decision-making process become even more difficult to define, process, and discuss. Consequently, in each single case, it is essential to evaluate and consider, from medical, legislative, and ethical points of view, the role of the "child/person" in the decision-making process that concerns them and the roles of the child's guardians/parents and care team.

Low patient numbers: Compared to adults/elderly patients receiving PC, the number of children eligible for PPC is much lower; this aspect, linked to the broad geographical distribution of patients, undeniably produces difficulties at organizational, training, skills, and costs levels.

A relatively recent event: Until a few years ago, most children who today are eligible for PPC would have died at birth or shortly after the diagnosis of their condition. Technological advances and the availability of new medical devices have led to a progressive and continuous increase in the number of children who live with serious illness for many years. These "recent cases" are still met with a severe lack of awareness and education, which generates shortcomings and barriers for those accessing care or organizing care solutions.

Emotional involvement: It is undeniable that a diagnosis of incurable illness and the death of a child are devastating and traumatic events for all those involved. The family members, distraught by grief, can lose their sense of purpose, modify their behavior, and become confused about their role, boundaries, and perspectives. Likewise for the healthcare workers called upon to address the child's complex needs, where professionalism, ethics, and deontology may conflict with their personal feelings, experiences, and fears. Regardless of their relationship with the child, these situations often incite reactions of anger, flight, or denial and are sometimes accompanied by unjustified and unrealistic faith in the curative abilities of medicine or a detached acceptance of the outcome. There is a serious risk of a disproportionate emotive reaction resulting in inappropriate invasive treatment or therapeutic abandonment.

All these issues combine to influence the types and entities of very particular needs that can only be met by implementing highly specific organizational decisions and patient care models.

Epidemiological Data

The range of conditions potentially eligible for PPC is heterogeneous and wide ranging: children with neurological, muscular, respiratory, metabolic, chromosomal, malformations, and post-anoxic conditions represent more than 60 percent of eligible patients. Fewer than 20 percent have cancer. Children with complex pathologies but without a well-defined diagnosis represent a considerable proportion of this population. Many conditions are rare, and some are genetically transmitted, with a possible multiple recurrence in siblings.

These illnesses frequently have a "wave-shaped" progression, characterized by unpredictable phases of remission alternating with phases of sudden intensification that requires emergency intervention and difficult treatment choices. These very challenging choices can greatly impact the child's quality of life or survival.

From a numerical point of view, the problem is certainly not to be underestimated. The WHO estimates that there are 21 million children worldwide with conditions for which there is no cure and for whom the only alternative treatment is PPC (Connor, Downing, & Marston, 2017; Rosenberg et al., 2019).

In Europe, the prevalence of children with pathologies eligible for PPC is significant and progressively increasing; a recent study in the United Kingdom estimated a prevalence of 32 cases per 10,000 children in 2009–2010, thus doubling the prevalence of 16 per 10,000 estimated in 2007. In Italy, a survey carried out in 2009 with very restrictive inclusion criteria showed that there were at least 12,000 children eligible for PPC (10 children out of 10,000).

Despite the ever-increasing need for PPC, unfortunately, in many parts of the world, the lack of services is still significant, and the healthcare solutions available are extremely limited. This shortfall is also evident in the European region, where PPC services are completely absent in one-third of the countries and where PPC is integrated into other healthcare services aimed at the child and family in only 12 percent of the countries.

There are numerous factors that have determined issues and obstructed the progression and introduction of PPC, causing an imbalance between patient needs and service provision. These are attributable to cultural, social, organizational, and economics causes but, above all else, to the lack of education and training (Twamley et al., 2014; Benini et al., 2016). The WHO invites the medical community to concentrate its efforts on this last couple of critical issues so that professional education, training, and social awareness can be the true driving forces of a much-needed and overdue change.

Addressing the Needs of Child and Family

To appropriately address the needs of the child and family, competent solutions to the multiplicity of clinical, social, psychological, organizational, spiritual, and ethical needs linked to serious illness and death must be foreseen.

Children's Needs

For the child, it is important to evaluate and address the following (Wolfe et al., 2018; European Association, 2007; Robert et al., 2019):

Clinical needs: Childhood illness very frequently engenders pain and neurological, respiratory, physiatrist, feeding, cognitive, and communication difficulties that impose multiple care solutions that encompass both symptom management and the use of technological management to support and monitor vital functions.

Psychological needs: In most cases, the children express a need to know and understand what is happening and what will happen to them in the short and long term. All the studies concur in affirming the importance of communication with the child: communication that must use instruments and strategies appropriate to their specific age, clinical situation, and cognitive development. It is important to create opportunities for the children to talk about their concerns and hopes and, at the same time, to reassure them that they will be supported and receive suitable care. It is essential to recognize and respect the child's role within a wide range of situations and their manner of communication. Additionally, it is important to perceive and interpret, with professionalism and competence, what the child conveys through a multiplicity of indirect messages, body language, and spoken words. Regrettably, regardless of the children's age and level of cognitive development, they are often treated as if they are unable to suffer and feel pain, incapable of asking questions about their illness and their future, not allowed to talk about their own wishes and concerns, or too young to participate in choices and decisions regarding their treatment. However, research, clinical experience, and everyday practice show us how wrong this concept is; it has, in fact, been demonstrated that all children, no matter how young or fragile, feel pain and experience all the clinical, emotional, psychological, and spiritual issues that serious illness and death entail and that, if listened to and supported, they are able to convey what they really want and what could help them the most.

The need for social integration and contact with peer groups: The integration of children and adolescents with serious illness within a social context (be it scholastic or friendship) begins and develops through the cultivation of a welcoming environment where mutual acceptance and respect of individual differences is fundamental. To achieve this goal, it is necessary to raise awareness in the social framework/network of friends and to communicate with the school to train educators how to include these children/adolescents in daily activities.

Spiritual needs: Throughout the course of the illness, it is essential to respect the cultural, social, and religious background of the child and family and maintain an open and accepting attitude toward the doubts and questions that they may express regarding the philosophical reasons for life, illness, and death.

In each individual case, the child's needs change constantly in intensity and prevalence linked to psychological, physical, and emotional development and the progression of the illness and its effects on the child's physical growth and cognitive development. However limited the child's life expectancy is and however severely affected or underdeveloped they may be, the acquisition of new functions and abilities is important. The child's growth and development are both core issues that must be at the center of any action undertaken – from the more traditional healthcare procedures (pharmacological treatments, supplementation or substitution of vital functions or organs, etc.) to those involving other aspects of society: the fostering of personal growth, education, cultural and creative inputs, spiritual support for the child and family, and upkeep of their role within the community.

Family Needs

The diagnosis of a child's incurable illness can have a traumatic effect on the whole family unit; their future prospects, roles, relationships, hopes, and beliefs are suddenly undermined. They encounter many stressful situations – from the emotional, psychological, social, and financial problems arising from the child's diagnosis to being responsible for providing the child's care and making important decisions in their best interests. The family is central to any PPC program, and they often bear the heavy social and financial burden of their child's illness, which, without adequate support, can be overwhelming.

The family's many needs include (Field & Behrman, 2003; European Association, 2007; Lazzarin, Schiavon, Brugnaro, & Benini, 2018):

Communication: This need is a priority that must be addressed in an honest, clear, welcoming, and respectful manner at all times and in any situation. It is fundamental to continually share clinical updates/care options and to recognize and respect the parents' choices through a dynamic and continuous dialogue where competence, time, respect, and mediation skills are the most effective tools for a correct valorization of roles. However, the responsibility of decision-making must not be delegated solely to the parents; choices must be shared and guided on the basis of what medical science can realistically achieve.

Psychological support: Parents require assessment, support, and treatment for feelings such as guilt, anger, depression, anticipatory grief, and denial. A child's illness can deeply undermine the family's stability, both at an individual level and as a couple. It can cause depression and a complete loss of their role or, alternatively, deep-seated anger and an inability to create constructive and cooperative relationships. If not supported properly, the rapport between couples becomes conflicting and stressful; they may become estranged and even separate. The families of children receiving PPC must be listened to and supported and their doubts, opinions, and anger acknowledged. They must be supported through their problems and plans and their silences, fears, and anxieties; even their desperation must be accepted.

Social and economic support: Family-centered home care is the goal of PPC, as it is what most children and families want and has a significant impact on their quality of life. However, home care is never a straightforward option, and the family must be supported. The burden of providing care is often considerable (estimated at almost nine hours per day) and determines important modifications to the family's daily routine. Very often one of the parents resigns from their workplace to care full-time for the child, while the other may move to a less challenging position and renounce any career expectations. This inevitably has a detrimental impact on the family's finances, on the family's social position, on the prospects of the individual parent, and on the family as a whole.

Training and empowerment: The family members must be provided with training in various aspects of patient care. Children receiving PPC frequently depend on devices and medical equipment for which it is important that family members receive training regarding use; they also need training on the management of crises and emergencies, as well as information on how to best reorganize their living space with consideration to the child's care and social needs.

Spiritual needs: Access to appropriate and competent spiritual support foreseeing an open exchange of ideas, doubts, and questions, in full respect of the family's cultural background and religious beliefs, is fundamental throughout the course of the child's illness and into bereavement.

Serious illness and the death of a child have devastating, long-term implications for the whole family. The child's siblings have a particular need of psychological support, as the experience may leave them feeling guilty or abandoned; they may also suffer from social isolation. They are considered at high risk of encountering problems at school and in their rapport with their parents, and they may also be prone to other psychological and social problems after their sibling's death. These problems are significantly reduced if their sibling is cared for at home rather than in a hospital.

Other members of the extended family (grandparents, uncles and aunts, and friends) can play an important part in sharing responsibilities and providing emotional support during the child's illness and after death; these individuals also need support and direction.

Care Team Needs

Together with the needs of children and families, it is important that the care team members' needs be evaluated and acknowledged. The care teams must deal with complex situations where the individuality and complexity of the child's care encounters the individuality and complexity of the personal tragedy of an incurable illness. These situations are far from being "simple"; in fact, they are nearly always difficult to conceive and experience from both professional and personal points of view. There are often circumstances that are difficult to accept, handle, and cope with as an integral part of life, illness, and treatment. The multiple care needs of these children and families can only be properly addressed by a multidisciplinary team; it is the team that evaluates each individual case and the impact of the illness on the patient and family, and together they discuss treatments, goals, and possible care options and establish strategies and care plans. Only through teamwork, through the collective discussion of critical issues and problems, is it possible for care team members to funnel their physiological emotions in a professional approach and so ensure effective and appropriate care provision.

The team needs include (Field & Behrman, 2003; Himelstein et al., 2004; European Association, 2007; Bergsträsser, Cignacco, & Luck, 2017):

Professional education and skills training: Several studies carried out among healthcare workers in Europe and the United States have highlighted an important lack of know-how regarding the fundamentals of palliative care delivery. Different types of knowledge are essential; in addition to the medical training essential for diagnosis and treatment, it is also necessary to be trained in communication strategies (with the child and family), teamwork, and in-service organization.

Support and supervision: The emotional impact and job stress involved in PPC delivery are undeniable and often are the cause of severe burnout in the care team members, which inevitably leads to a rapid turnover of staff and adverse implications for human and economic resources. To break this cycle and to help them cope with the difficulties of caring for patients with incurable illness, the care team must be supported, listened to, and supervised so that they can continue to care competently for patients without becoming overly physically and emotionally drained.

Resources: Until recently, PPC provision was not considered a fundamental healthcare service, and the expertise of clinicians working in this field was barely acknowledged. Today, the situation is changing; it has been demonstrated in numerous research studies and is widely recognized in daily clinical practice that PPC is a fundamental aspect of healthcare delivery and necessitates the allocation of specific funding, as service provision is currently far from adequate and is failing to meet patient needs.

Public awareness: The general public needs to be better informed about PC and to consider access to PC services, which safeguards the quality of life, dignity, and personal identity of the most vulnerable members of our society when they are seriously ill and dying, as a basic human right.

If the general public, patients, and their families are well informed of what is available and how services are accessible, this can facilitate the work of care teams; it enables cooperation, the resolution of difficulties, and the identification of strategies to best address everyone's needs.

Healthcare Models

Due to the nature of the conditions involved and to the multiplicity and intensity of related care needs, care provision for these children encounters clinical and organizational barriers that are not easy to overcome. From an epidemiological point of view, the prevalence of these pathologies is relatively rare, and they have a broad geographical distribution. At the same time, each case is distinct and presents a multiplicity of clinical, psychological, and social needs that necessitate care delivery managed by a specialist team and concurrently from a series of healthcare agencies and institutions all within reasonable distance of the child's home. Care must be available continuously, even over prolonged periods (months or years), and must address complex needs that, depending on the progression of the illness, are in continuous evolution both in prevalence and intensity and directly linked to the child's psycho-physical-emotional development (Rusalen, Agosto, Brugraro, & Benini, 2017; Chong, De Castro Molina, Teo, & Tan, 2018; Zernikow et al., 2019; Vadeboncoeur & Mchardy, 2018).

The care model capable of addressing the numerous issues related to PPC delivery, indicated in numerous studies and proposed in many international PPC programs, is the organization of dedicated, child-specific PC networks covering large areas (usually a geographic region) that are coordinated from a reference center by a specialized multidisciplinary care team (Mherekumombe, 2018; Grunauer & Mikesell, 2018). The team works in unison with the local healthcare agencies and social services to provide effective, continuous care and support for the child and family (see Figure 15.1).

The aim of the network is to ensure multifaceted, specialized, continuous care as near as possible to the child's usual environment, ideally in the family home. The network, overseen by the PPC reference center, offers flexible and constant care across a series of care settings (residential and in home)

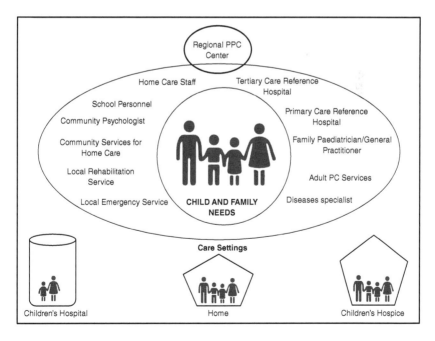

Figure 15.1 Pediatric Palliative Care Networks Model.

that can be accessed at any time according to the child's and family's needs. The network encompasses all of the local healthcare agencies/organizations/institutions involved in the child's care and pools and cooperates with all the healthcare networks, pediatric and other, operating in the area. The PPC reference center, which is usually the seat of the children's hospice, acts as a pivot for the supervision of the clinical, organizational, training, and research processes linked to the network operations. It is also responsible for the development, organization, evaluation, and monitoring of all procedural aspects. The center identifies training and communication needs for the network's catchment area and implements strategies and initiatives for caregiver training and public information campaigns.

Although family-centered home care is the goal of PPC and is, in most cases, what the child and family want and has a positive impact on their quality of life; sometimes, however, because of procedural or clinical complications linked to the child's condition, fatigue, emotional stress, or perhaps logistic and organizational difficulties, care delivery in the family home is not possible. In these cases, a temporary residential solution is essential, and the children's hospice, as an alternative to hospitalization, offers the most appropriate solution. Presenting elevated diagnostic and therapeutic competences, it facilitates the activation of effective and integrated home-care programs involving all the components of the network, and, at the same time, it is a child-centered environment with areas, rooms, furnishings, and an organization tailored to their needs in a setting very similar to that of a family home.

In diverse contexts (systems, geographical, resource), this network model may present some subtle differences; however, there are several organizational aspects that are high priority: the provision of separate child-specific networks (not integrated with services for adults or older people), centralized care coordination, and continuous care/support available 24/7.

In the regions where PPC reference centers and networks are operational, the outcomes are very positive – from a reduction in inappropriate hospitalizations of children with complex pathologies to an improved perception of healthcare delivery and, above all, enhanced quality of life of the children and their families (Rusalen et al., 2017; Chong et al., 2018; Zernikow et al., 2019; Vadeboncoeur & Mchardy, 2018).

Conclusions

The current lack of PPC provision is not an easy problem to resolve due to the broad scope of skills and resources necessary for the implementation of efficient and realistic care solutions. However, effective strategies to resolve this cultural, organizational, and healthcare challenge are persistently coming to the forefront in leading scientific publications, where training, raised awareness, and research are confirmed as the essential actions to be undertaken for a long-overdue transformation in care delivery for children living with serious illness (Rosenberg & Wolfe, 2017; Slater et al., 2018; Weaver et al., 2019; Brand McCarthy, Kang, & Mack, 2019; Decourcey, Silverman, Oladunjoye, & Wolfe, 2019; Field & Behrman, 2003; National Guideline Alliance, 2016; Loeffen et al., 2018; Lotz, Daxer, Jox, Borasio, & Führer, 2017; Benini et al., 2017).

From an *organizational viewpoint*, early access to PPC services and a continual dialogue regarding individual care goals, options, strategies, and programs, together with sustained staff training, raised social awareness, clear guidelines, and proficiencies in legal and ethical questions most certainly enhance the care provided for these children. Effective PPC provision greatly impacts their quality of life and death, which, in turn, has long-term implications for the well-being and mental health of family members, particularly siblings.

Purely from a *viewpoint of healthcare provision* for the child and family, the following must be considered priorities:

- To re-establish, contextualize, and divulge that the actual goal of care delivery is the child's well-being, where well-being is understood in a "global" sense and not just limited to symptom control and/or the recovery of a bodily function and/or system without due consideration of the physical, cognitive, and social person of which that symptom or function is a part. With the child's well-being as the care goal, all choices, decisions, and actions must be undertaken accordingly. "Doing everything that is technically possible" is contextualized in PPC as "doing everything that the situation requires." All options and choices must be contemplated within the limits of medical science, and, in full understanding of these limits, the best possible care that medical science can realistically offer should be provided.
- To practice competence and professionalism in order to promote a constant and consistent dialogue with the children and their families; the aim is to build a reliable, honest, nonjudgmental, supportive, and accepting rapport with them.
- To acknowledge and respect the child's role in the full scope of their diversity and be conscious of their methods of communication and to acknowledge and respect the parents' role.
- To constantly share information regarding the clinical situation and care choices with all the members of the multi-professional care team in order to propose consistent care options based on feasible therapeutic procedures, clinical experience, and shared expert decisions.

These are all situations that induce questions and reflections regarding the meaning of life and of human existence, interrogations that go beyond the boundaries of medicine but that must not only receive appropriate and competent answers but must also be addressed on social, cultural, ethical, and legislative levels, aspects that must be mediated by a responsible "humanity."

Palliative Care in the Elderly

Ferdinando Cancelli, MD

A.L. is 74 years old. She has been suffering from Parkinson's disease for five years, and the clinical situation is getting worse. She is assisted at home by her 77-year-old husband, still in good health. Despite an increased dosage of levodopa and the use of pramipexole, muscle rigidity is increasing, walking is getting more uncertain, and daily activities are increasingly compromised. There is also a progressive psychic impairment with a depressive anxiety syndrome that is difficult to control despite antidepressant therapy, and at certain times, it's difficult for her to leave the house. The husband is in difficulty, despite having renounced any type of activity outside the home and devoted himself to his wife all day; it is increasingly hard to cover the needs of care. The children, now adults, both work and have not been at home for years. Their modest financial resources do not allow the couple to hire a caregiver, and in case of further deterioration, it could be necessary for A.L. to stay in a nursing home. The national health system offers little economic aid, and finding a nursing home is very difficult and involves high costs. Prospects for the future when A.L. will no longer be able to swallow properly will be incontinence and her being bound to a wheelchair or in bed, events that are scaring the couple.

The case of this patient is more and more frequent in the clinical practice of palliative care for elderly patients. This chapter will try to answer the following questions, which apply to A.L. as well as many other individuals:

- What is the advanced age situation in Western countries?
- What does it mean to integrate palliative care and geriatrics care?
- Which diseases and symptoms most frequently require palliative care in the elderly?
- What are the most frequent settings and care paths?
- What pharmacological and clinical peculiarities does the elderly patient show?
- Advance care planning and end-of-life choices: what awareness do patients have?

Advanced Age and Demographic Changes

Societies, particularly in Western countries, are aging (World Health Organization, 2015). The percentage of the population over 65 years of age, which by definition we consider "old," is steadily growing. Today in the European Union (EU), a 50-year-old male has a life expectancy of 29 years and a 50-year-old woman of about 34 years. But of these years, only about 10 will be free of morbidity (Jagger et al., 2011; Voumard, 2018). The fact is impressive even if compared with the situation in United States: in 1900, life expectancy at birth was less than 50 years.

In the EU in 2009, 15 percent of the population was over 65, particularly in the Mediterranean countries. By 2050, this percentage will rise to more than 25 percent, and the biggest increase will be for people over 85 (OECD Factbook, 2009). The number of nonagenarians was 1.9 million in 2010, and that number is expected to quadruple by 2050 in United States (Chai, Meier, Morris, & Goldhirsch, 2014).

The needs of the elderly therefore increase at various levels with respect to prevention, care, quality of life, and good conditions of death. The entire society is involved, and first and foremost are the patients, caregivers, national health systems, politics, and universities. And if this is true for palliative care directed at all ages, starting from pediatric patients, it is even more true for geriatric palliative care.

Recently in this regard and to promote diffusion and correct implementation of palliative care worldwide, a "White Book" was published by the Pontifical Academy for Life with a series of recommendations made by an expert advisory group and directed to policymakers, universities, healthcare workers, hospitals, palliative care associations, international organizations, mass media, pharmacists, and others stakeholders all over the world (PAL-LIFE, 2019).

The Definition of Palliative Care and the Geriatric Approach

Geriatrics is the branch of medicine that deals with the diagnosis and treatment of diseases and problems specific for elderly (American Geriatric Society).

With respect to palliative care, the Lancet Commission on Global Access to Palliative Care and Pain Relief published a report, *Alleviating the Access Abyss in Palliative Care and Pain Relief – An Imperative of Universal Health Coverage* (Knaul et al., 2018). The new approach by the commission resulted in a broader concept of palliative care, more suitable for addressing the burden of chronic diseases and serious health-related suffering. Following the recommendations of the commission, the International Association for Hospice and Palliative Care (IAHPC) developed and implemented a project to revise the definition for palliative care. The first section of the definition says: "Palliative care is the active holistic care of individuals across all ages with serious health-related suffering due to severe illness, and especially of those near the end of life. It aims to improve the quality of life of patients, their families and their caregivers."

Palliative care:

• Includes prevention, early identification, comprehensive assessment, and management of physical issues, including pain and other distressing symptoms, psychological distress, spiritual distress, and social needs. Whenever possible, these interventions must be evidence based.

- Provides support to help patients live as fully as possible until death by facilitating effective communication, helping them and their families determine goals of care.
- Is applicable throughout the course of an illness, according to the patient's needs.
- Is provided in conjunction with disease-modifying therapies whenever needed.
- May positively influence the course of illness.
- Intends neither to hasten nor postpone death, affirms life, and recognizes dying as a natural process.
- Provides support to the family and the caregivers during the patient's illness and in their own bereavement.
- Is delivered recognizing and respecting the cultural values and beliefs of the patient and the family.
- Is applicable throughout all healthcare settings (place of residence and institutions) and in all levels (primary to tertiary).
- Can be provided by professionals with basic palliative care training.
- Requires specialist palliative care with a multiprofessional team for referral of complex cases.

Some points of the new definition are particularly important for geriatric palliative care:

- In the second section of the definition, it is specified that it is necessary to "Ensure access to adequate palliative care for vulnerable groups, including children and older persons."
- It is specified that palliative care takes care of individuals of all ages.
- Not only the end-of-life phase but also the earliest stages of illness can benefit from a palliative approach. If we think of nononcological degenerative diseases such as dementia or Parkinson's disease, it is clear that these early and intermediate stages of the disease can be very long and burdened with important symptoms. Palliative care for elders differs from what is usually appropriate for younger adults due to the nature and duration of chronic illness during old age.
- Palliative care aims to improve the quality of life of patients and also of their families and caregivers.
- Palliative care does not accelerate or delay death at all costs. Compared to elderly patients for whom, on the one hand, the risk is one of disproportionate therapies and, on the other, of excessive abstention, it is important to reiterate what is already present in the WHO definition.
- Palliative care is applicable throughout healthcare settings: older adults often make multiple transitions across care settings, especially in the last months of life, and therefore it is important to ensure that care plans and patients' goals are preserved from one setting to another (Morrison, 2013).

Geriatric palliative care combines the approach of these two specialties and is based on the following shared core principles (Chai et al., 2014): clarifying and documenting individual and family preferences and goals of care; providing care that is patient and family centered and evidence based; employing an interdisciplinary team approach; giving careful attention to medication management; using interpersonal and communication skills that result in effective information exchange with patients, their families, and other health professionals; coordinating care; respecting the importance of family caregivers and recognizing and addressing their needs; maximizing quality of life and functionality; providing psychosocial, spiritual, and bereavement support to patients and caregivers; and delivering ethical care that is aligned with patient and family preferences and that always balances the benefits and burden of therapeutic interventions.

Palliative Care in the Elderly: Diseases and Symptoms

Very often elderly patients have multiple chronic degenerative diseases, even evolving simultaneously. There are not infrequent cases of elderly cancer patients in whom diseases such as heart disease, chronic renal failure, diabetes, and/or chronic obstructive pulmonary disease coexist. One-quarter of people aged 85 years and older have dementia (Ferri et al., 2005). This justifies a palliative and geriatric approach during all phases of the disease, as defined by the IAHPC, and allows us to understand why palliative care is a part of the curriculum for training in geriatric medicine recommended in the EU (Geriatric Medicine Section) and why better integration among palliative, primary, and social care is of paramount importance.

The main causes of death are, in decreasing order, ischemic heart disease, cerebrovascular disease (including stroke), chronic obstructive pulmonary disease, lower respiratory infections, and cancer (World Health Organization, 2004). The incidence and prevalence of various disturbing physical symptoms has been investigated, especially in cancer patients (Van Lancker et al., 2014; Morita et al., 2014), and the main symptoms described are fatigue, with a prevalence of almost 80 percent of patients, followed by various palliative care teams; urinary incontinence, with a prevalence of more than 70 percent; asthenia (66.7 percent), pain (66.3 percent); constipation (52.5 percent); dyspnea (55 percent); and anxiety and psychic symptoms (50 percent). Other not less burdensome physical symptoms are, for example, coughing, hiccups, itching, and insomnia. It should be noted that syndromes affecting older people who are not included in palliative care textbooks, such as urinary incontinence and falls, can badly compromise the quality of life for patients and families (World Health Organization, 2011).

A very particular situation is represented by dementia, an incurable disease at present. The prognosis can range from 2 to more than 15 years, with the end stage lasting as long as 2 to 3 years; there are 4.6 million new cases every year worldwide (Ferri et al., 2005; World Health Organization, 2011). Many studies affirm that the number of people with dementia is predicted to double every 20 years. Most people with dementia in medium and advanced stages need 24-hour care for cognitive, functional, and physical impairment (McCarthy, Addington-Hall, & Altman, 1997). Geriatric palliative care should have the role of avoiding many disproportionate interventions (tube feeding, laboratory tests, use of restraints) and of guaranteeing better control of symptoms, often undertreated; better support for caregivers; and a global and holistic approach to the patient. The difficulty of making a precise prognostic judgment is one of the reasons people do not receive adequate palliative care: often healthcare professionals do not perceive people with dementia as having a terminal condition (Small, 2007). For this reason, when possible, advance care planning must be initiated at a very early stage.

Particular attention in a palliative care setting should be paid to pain and its management in the elderly patient. Several studies have shown that pain is in many cases insufficiently controlled in older people because they tend to trivialize the pain as a normal condition of age, but also because the caregivers can underestimate the pain. All analgesics can be used in the elderly person with the condition of starting at low doses, taking into account renal function and malnutrition, and then titrating the increase in doses according to the analgesic effect obtained and the side effects (Pautex & Vogt-Ferrier, 2006). An evaluation of pain should be done systematically in all elderly patients given the high prevalence of pain in this age group. Numeric rating scales (NRSs), verbal descriptor scales (VDSs), face pain scales (FPSs), and visual analogue scales (VASs) are appropriate for use with older adults (Keela & Garand, 2001), provided that doctors or nurses take time to explain to the patient and to choose the one that is adapted to the possible hearing or vision disorders that can reduce comprehension in the elderly patient. The McGill Pain Questionnaire (MPQ) is a well-known tool for the thorough evaluation of pain location, intensity, temporal qualities, and sensitivity to change, as well as sensory and affective aspects of pain. Scales like Doloplus or Algoplus are widely used in Francophone countries for the evaluation of pain in the elderly (Rostad, Utne, Grov, Puts, & Halvorsrud, 2017).

As will be explained later, the pharmacokinetics of drugs is modified by advancing age. Thus, the volume of distribution of water-soluble and fat-soluble drugs is modified, and the cardiac, hepatic, and renal rates decrease. Malnutrition has various effects on pharmacokinetics: it may be accompanied by a small body weight with risk of overdose at standard dose by altering the total volume of distribution, alteration of the distribution phase due to proportional changes in different compartments of the body, and finally hypoalbuminemia. The introduction of a drug strongly bound to albumin (for example, bromazepam) in the presence of other drugs can then lead, especially at the beginning of treatment, to a high concentration of the active-free fraction of drug. Thus, elderly patients are subject to large interindividual variations in drug distribution and metabolism. They are at risk of accumulating drugs and having more drug interactions.

Drug doses eliminated by the kidney with a narrow therapeutic margin must be adapted (Pautex & Vogt-Ferrier, 2006). Given the high risk of drug interactions, prodrugs such as codeine should be avoided, dosage adjustments should be made, and attention should be paid to additive side effects such as drowsiness, confused states, or serotoninergic syndrome. An elderly patient who takes six medications is 14 times more likely to have a side effect than a younger person with the same number of medications (Rollason, Bonnabry, & Vogt, 2000). Nonopioids or first-step drugs of the WHO scale are the first-line treatments for mild to moderate pain. Paracetamol is the treatment of choice because of its relatively safe profile in elderly patients. Despite the fact that NSAIDs can be extremely useful in certain situations (for example, bone pain for metastases), care should be taken when administering them to the elderly, particularly in diabetic, hypertensive, or heart failure patients. Short-half-life NSAIDs are preferable (ibuprofen or diclofenac, for example) and should be prescribed for a period of time as short as possible. The third-step analgesics tend to be underutilized in elderly patients. However, morphine remains the opiate of reference for moderate to severe pain. The oral route should be preferred, and a titration is compulsory at the beginning of the treatment.

Most Frequent Settings and Care Paths

Although in our daily practice of palliative care we note a strong desire of patients to be treated at home and to die at home, even today most patients die in hospitals or nursing homes (Higginson & Sen-Gupta, 2000). Undoubtedly the social change in Western societies increases the difficulty of organizing assistance at home by finding helpful caregivers. More and more patients are living alone, there are more and more broken families, and fewer and fewer children have time to follow sick parents. Even though implementing home care could reduce the costs of assistance, national health systems struggle to find adequate solutions, especially in cases of chronic degenerative diseases with long prognosis. Recent Italian work has shown that globally around 65 percent of deaths occur in a medical facility and only 35 percent at home. Other countries have even lower home death rates: about half a million people die in England each year. Most deaths (58 percent) occur at National Health Service hospitals, with about 18 percent occurring at home, 17 percent in care homes, 4 percent in hospices, and 3 percent elsewhere (Chai et al., 2014).

In France, a law "on old age and autonomy" will be promulgated by the end of 2019. The law aims to encourage taking care of elderly patients at home. The "choices" of families are often strongly conditioned by economic conditions, and often taking care of elderly at home is very difficult due to lack of caregivers.

Concerning this, the National Observatory of the End of Life (Observatoire National de la Fin de la Vie, ONFV) published in France the report "End of Life of the Elderly: Seven Ordinary Paths to Better Understand End-of-Life Issues in France" (2013). The report tries to answer a few questions on the subject and, in particular, how seniors end their lives, what they do, and where and how they live when they reach this last period, where the border is between "old age" and the end of life, and if the expression "to die of old age" still has a meaning.

The study focuses on people whose daily lives are impacted by the consequences of aging and whose diseases are marked by specific end-of-life care needs. The analysis is done on different "end-of-life paths" to better meet the needs of a population affected by several diseases and who must move from one place of care to another.

The three main end-of-life trajectories are:

- Slow decline (e.g., cognitive disorders such as Alzheimer's disease), 10 percent of cases
- Gradual decline (e.g., organ failures such as heart failure, respiratory failure, kidney failure), 40 percent of cases
- Rapid decline (e.g., cancer), 50 percent of cases

Slow Decline (Cognitive Disorders Such as Alzheimer's Disease)

The three most important common points of slow decline trajectories are a late identification of the palliative situation; the exhaustion of caregivers, especially at home; and the multiplication of needs.

According to the report, about 38,000 people each year die in France from cognitive disorders; of these, 11,400 die in nursing homes for dependent elderly and 15,000 in hospital. In nursing homes, only 36 percent of residents have designated a person of trust (proxy) and 5 percent have drafted advance directives, even if the report notes progress in the field of pain relief and the application of French law on the end of life. More than a quarter of the residents die without being surrounded by their loved ones.

Depression remains underdiagnosed even in institutions; too often we forget that depression is in no way a consequence of normal aging. Suicide remains an important cause of death for the elderly person. In France in 2010, 2873 people older than 65 years ended their days (30 percent of total suicides). In the older than 85 years group, the prevalence of suicide is twice as high as that of the 25–44 age group, and men older than 95 years of age kill themselves on average 10 times more than the general population. More than 68 percent of these suicides take place at the person's home.

Gradual Decline (Organ Failure Such as Heart Failure, Respiratory Failure, Renal Failure)

The three most important common points of gradual decline trajectories are a lack of anticipation of complications related to the end of life; emergency management not adapted to the reality of a person's needs; and a lack of planning regarding the return to home from nursing homes, hospices, or hospitals, with a high rate of emergency rehospitalization.

Ninety percent of the elderly receive the intervention of a paid caregiver, a low-skilled job in France and in general in the EU; these caregivers often cope with the end of life, and 46 percent of carers are concerned about the end of life of the person they care for. They sometimes have great difficulty in recognizing the end of life, and they are very rarely trained.

Nearly 13,000 elderly people die each year in emergencies, and 61 percent of patients who died in the emergency department in 2010 were over 80 years old. Emergency services are not adapted to accommodate and accompany end-of-life situations and rarely palliative care is implemented. In 78.8 percent of cases, a decision to withdraw treatment was made by a doctor alone and without collegiality or patient consensus because of unconsciousness.

Rapid Decline (Cancer)

The three most important points of rapid decline trajectories are that often the patient spends his or her last months of life in the hospital, disproportionate treatments, and the difficulty of the decision-making process at the end of life. About 155,000 people die of cancer every year in France, but sometimes the palliative orientation is very late and the preparation of the return home is very insufficient, with high rates of rehospitalization after discharge.

More than 49 percent of people who die of cancer in the hospital spent their last month of life there, with 73 percent of cancer deaths occurring in the hospital. In the last week before death, nearly half of patients in the hospital received treatment for acute episodes.

Last, few French people have designated their "trusted person": about 25 percent of end-of-life patients have made a decision to limit or discontinue treatment. Only 1.5 percent of patients concerned had drafted their advance directives.

The ONFV report clearly shows the weak points of assistance to elderly people at the end of the life and during their illness. Many challenges are in front of us at the moment and for the future.

Pharmacological and Clinical Peculiarities of Elderly Patients: Less Is More

In 2005, CAD$24.8 billion were spent in Canada on drugs, of which 44 percent were prescribed to those aged 65 years and older (Canada Institute for Health Information, 2005). According to Marengoni et al. (2011), the number of "oldest old" people will reach 75 million in 2060 in Europe and will consume more and more drugs.

The palliative care approach tends to prescribe the drugs strictly neces-sary for the control of physical and mental symptoms, giving preference to the oral route of administration when possible and minimizing invasive interventions. Prescription of drugs is a fundamental component of the care of elderly people, particularly of those at the end of the life (Spinewine et al., 2007). Furthermore, elderly people have several comorbidities, asso-ciated polymedication ("polypharmacy" defined as the chronic intake of five or more drugs) (Mannucci, Nobili, & Pasina, 2018), age-related impair-ments in the hepatic metabolism and renal clearance, and enhanced phar-macodynamic sensitivity to specific drugs (Mangoni & Jackson, 2004). In some cases, especially in advanced stages of disease, they might not main-tain adequate nutritional status. For these reasons, inappropriate prescrib-ing can cause substantial morbidity and represent a clinical and economic burden to patients and society. Prescribing should aim to promote the use of evidence-based therapies and keep the use of drugs for which there is no clinical need or where there is dubious efficacy to a minimum (Spinewine et al., 2007).

Some of the more frequent drug interactions in elderly patients can be drug–drug pharmacokinetic interactions (e.g., ciprofloxacin and olanzapine: cipro-floxacin inhibits CYP1A2, leading to an increase in plasma concentration of olanzapine that leads to rigidity and falls, particularly in patients with Parkin-son's disease) (Spinewine et al., 2007), drug–drug pharmacodynamic interac-tion (e.g., ciprofloxacin and glibenclamide: the synergy can lead to profound hypoglycemia), drug–nutritional status interaction (e.g., low albumin and phe-nytoin with increase in phenytoin concentration and confusion, somnolence, and ataxia), drug–herbal product interaction (e.g., ginkgo and aspirin: decrease in platelet function and adhesion with increased risk of bleeding), and drug–alcohol interaction and drug–disease interaction (e.g., metoclopramide for gas-tric dysmotility in a patient with Parkinson's disease: increase in dopamine receptor blockade with worsening Parkinson's disease). In a European study of 1601 elderly outpatients, 46 percent of patients had at least one potential clini-cally significant drug–drug interaction, and 10 percent of these interactions were regarded as high severity (Bjorkman et al., 2002). Consider what effects the simple administration of an antibiotic such as ciprofloxacin can have in an already fragile patient.

We can affirm that the "deprescribing" (Scott et al., 2015) – defined as the systematic process of identifying and discontinuing drugs in instances in which existing or potential harms outweigh existing or potential benefits within the context of an individual patient's care goals, current level of functioning, life expectancy, values, and preferences – should be a current practice in palliative care. Particular precautions must also be taken in prescribing pain medication: avoiding NSAIDs, prescribing the minimum effective doses of opioids such as morphine, and preferring opioids best suited for renal failure such as transder-mal fentanyl.

End-of-Life Choices and Aging

Advanced age is characterized by a particular fragility: the many diseases and the conditions of dependence and loneliness in which the elderly find themselves are likely to make the last years of life very hard. In Western societies, increasingly marked by activism and health fanaticism, the elderly are inclined to feel a burden on others: no longer productive, often unable to keep up with the changes in digitalization, they often are the first victims of a new form of social marginalization. In addition to this, the loneliness of elderly patients plays against them; families are increasingly reduced and, especially in large cities, the elderly who are unable to take care of themselves find themselves increasingly alone.

In 2016, the Dutch government announced its intention to recognize existential suffering by itself as a valid ground for assisted suicide, especially for elderly people over a certain age who have "completed lives." The concept of unbearable suffering, as well explained by John Keown, is expanding from suffering while living to suffering from living (2018). A survey of the attitudes of elderly Dutch people in 2012 found that an increasing proportion could imagine asking for a suicide if they were tired of life in the absence of a severe disease (Buiting et al., 2012); another survey in 2015 disclosed that 36 percent of respondents agreed that "the oldest old should be able to get medications that enable them, if they wish, to end their life," and 21 percent agreed that "euthanasia should be allowed for people who are tired of living, without having a serious disease" (Raijmakers et al., 2015). In 2004, the Dijkhuis Committee in the Netherlands expressed its support for "suffering from life," which it defined as "suffering at the prospect of having to continue living in a manner in which there is not only a deficient, perceived quality of life, giving rise to a persisting desire to die, even though the absence or deficiency in quality of life cannot be explained in any or significant measure by an identifiable somatic or psychological condition" (KNMG, 2011).

In this regard, the concept of "quality of life" can be a double-edged sword. Made with the intent to improve the living conditions of patients, its use can incite some patients, consciously or not, to feel themselves to be a burden on others and to consider their life no longer worth living. In our medical experience, forcing the patient to face his own weaknesses by means of a questionnaire does not always prove to be helpful, and the use of quality-of-life questionnaires must be carefully evaluated case by case without becoming a routine means of evaluation.

In our opinion, palliative care, both at home and in hospice, is a powerful way to prevent elderly patients from feeling useless and burdensome for others when they reach the end of their lives. Assisted suicide or euthanasia claims in palliative care units are the lowest in hospitals. Referring to the hospice where I work, one of our patients one day told us: "I like this place because death, when it arrives, still finds us alive!"

Discussion Questions

1. How does palliative care differ in pediatrics versus aging?
2. How do palliative care physicians approach dying with dignity for children?

References

American Geriatric Society. (2012). *Guiding Principles for the Care of Older Adults with Multimorbidity: An Approach for Clinicians*. New York: Author.

Benini, F., Orzalesi, M., de Santi, A., Congedi, S., Lazzarin, P., Pellegatta, F., . . . Alleva, E. (2016). Barriers to the development of pediatric palliative care in Italy. *Annali dell'Istituto Superiore di Sanità* 52(4), 558–564. doi:10.4415/ANN_16_04_16.

Benini, F., Vecchi, R., Lazzarin, P., Jankovic, M., Orsi, L., Manfredini, L., . . . Orzalesi, M. (2017, January). The rights of the dying child and the duties of healthcare providers: The "Trieste Charter". *Tumori* 103(1), 33–39. doi:10.5301/tj.5000566.

Bergsträsser, E., Cignacco, E., & Luck, P. (2017, August). Health care professionals' experiences and needs when delivering end-of-life care to children: A qualitative study. *Palliative Care* 10. doi:10.1177/1178224217724770.

Bjorkman, I. K., et al. (2002). Drug-drug interactions in the elderly. *Annals of Pharmacotherapy* 36, 1675–1681.

Brand McCarthy, S. R., Kang, T. I., & Mack, J. W. (2019, April). Inclusion of children in the initial conversation about their cancer diagnosis: Impact on parent experiences of the communication process. *Supportive Care in Cancer* 27(4), 1319–1324. doi:10.1007/s00520-019-4653-3.

Buiting, H. M., Deeg, D. J., Knol, D. L., Ziegelmann, J. P., Pasman, H. R., & Widdershoven, G. A., et al. (2012). Older people's attitudes towards euthanasia and an end-of-life pill in the Netherlands: 2001–2009. *Journal of Medical Ethics* 38, 267.

Canadian Institute for Health Information. (2005). *National Health Expenditure Trends 1975 to 2005*. Ottawa: National Health Expenditure Database.

Chai, E., Meier, D., Morris, J., & Goldhirsch, S. (2014). *Geriatric Palliative Care*. Oxford: Oxford University Press.

Chong, P. H., De Castro Molina, J. A., Teo, K., & Tan, W. S. (2018, January). Paediatric palliative care improves patient outcomes and reduces healthcare costs: Evaluation of a home-based program. *BMC Palliative Care* 17(1), 11. doi:10.1186/s12904-017-0267-z.

Connor, S. R., Downing, J., & Marston, J. (2017, February). Estimating the global need for palliative care for children: A cross-sectional analysis. *Journal of Pain and Symptom Management* 53(2), 171–177. doi:10.1016/j.jpainsymman.2016.08.020.

DeCourcey, D. D., Silverman, M., Oladunjoye, A., & Wolfe, J. (2019, January). Advance care planning and parent-reported end-of-life outcomes in children, adolescents, and young adults with complex chronic conditions. *Critical Care Medicine* 47(1), 101–108. doi:10.1097/CCM.0000000000003472.

European Association of Palliative Care (EAPC) Taskforce. (2007). IMPaCCT: Standards for paediatric palliative care in Europe. *European Journal of Palliative Care* 14, 2–7.

Ferri, C. P., Prince, M., Brayne, C., Brodaty, H., Fratiglioni, L., Ganguli, M., Hall, K., . . . Scazufca, M. (2005). Global prevalence of dementia: A Delphi consensus study. *Lancet* 366, 2112–2117.

Field, M. J., & Behrman, R. E. (Eds.). (2003). *When Children Die: Improving Palliative and End-of-Life Care for Children and Their Families*. Washington, DC: National Academies Press.

Friedrichsdorf, S. J., & Bruera, E. (2018, August 31). Delivering pediatric palliative care: From denial, palliphobia, pallilalia to palliactive. *Children* (Basel) 5(9), E120. doi:10.3390/children5090120.

Geriatric Medicine Section, European Union of Medical Specialists. (1999). *Training in Geriatric Medicine in the European Union*. Brussels: European Union of Medical Specialists.

Goldman, A., Hain, R., & Liben, S. (2012). *Oxford Textbook of Palliative Care for Children*. Oxford: Oxford University Press.

Grunauer, M., & Mikesell, C. A. (2018, January). Review of the integrated model of care: An opportunity to respond to extensive palliative care needs in pediatric intensive care units in under-resourced settings. *Frontiers in Pediatrics* 6, 3. doi:10.3389/fped.2018.00003.

Higginson, I. J., & Sen-Gupta, G. J. A. (2000). Place of care in advanced cancer: A qualitative systematic literature review of patient preferences. *Journal of Palliative Medicine* 3, 287–300.

Himelstein, B. P., Hilden, J. M., Boldt, A. M., & Weissman, D. (2004). Pediatric palliative care. *New England Journal of Medicine* 350, 1752–1762.

Jagger, C., Weston, C., Cambois, E., Van Oyen, H., Nusselder, W., Doblhammer, G., . . . Robine, J.-M. (2011). Inequalities in health expectancies at older ages in European Union: Finding from the survey of health and retirement in Europe (SHARE). *Journal of Epidemiology and Community Health* 65(11), 1030–1035.

Keela, A., & Garand, L. (2001, August). Assessment and measurement of pain in older adults. *Clinical Geriatric Medicine* 17(3), 457 – 478.

Keown, J. (2018). *Euthanasia, Ethics and Public Policy*, 26. Cambridge: Cambridge University Press.

Knaul, F. M., Farmer, P., Krakauer, E., De Lima, L., Bhadelia, A., Kwete, X. J., . . . Rajagopal, M. R. (2018, April 7). Alleviating the access abyss in palliative care and pain relief: An imperative of universal health coverage. *Lancet* 391(10128), 1391–1454.

KNMG (Royal Dutch Medical Association). (2011, June). *The Role of the Physician in the Voluntary Termination of Life*. Utrecht: Author.

Lazzarin, P., Schiavon, B., Brugnaro, L., & Benini, F. (2018, February). Parents spend an average of nine hours a day providing palliative care for children at home and need to maintain an average of five life-saving devices. *Acta Paediatrica* 107(2), 289–293. doi:10.1111/apa.14098.

Loeffen, E. A. H., Tissing, W. J. E., Schuiling-Otten, M. A., de Kruiff, C. C., Kremer, L. C. M., & Verhagen, A. A. E. (2018). Pediatric Palliative Care – Individualized Care Plan Working Group: Individualised advance care planning in children with life-limiting conditions. *Archives of Disease in Childhood* 103(5), 480. doi:10.1136/archdischild-2017-312731.

Lotz, J. D., Daxer, M., Jox, R. J., Borasio, G. D., & Führer, M. (2017). "Hope for the best, prepare for the worst": A qualitative interview study on parents' needs and fears in pediatric advance care planning. *Palliative Medicine* 31(8), 764. doi:10.1177/0269216316679913.

Mangoni, A. A., & Jackson, S. H. (2004). Age-related changes in pharmacokinetics and pharmacodynamics: basic principles and practical applications. *British Journal of Clinical Pharmacology* 57, 6–14.

Mannucci, P. M., Nobili, A., & Pasina, L. (2018, August). Polypharmacy in older people: Lessons from 10 years of experience with the REPOSI register. *Internal and
Emergency Medicine* 13(8), 1191–1200.

Marengoni, A., Angleman, S., Melis, R., Mangialasche, F., Karp, A., Garmen, A., . . .
Fratiglioni, L. (2011). Aging with multimorbidity: A systematic review of the literature. *Ageing Research Reviews* 10, 430–439.

McCarthy, M., Addington-Hall, J., & Altman, D. (1997). The experience of dying with
dementia: A retrospective study. *International Journal of Geriatric Psychiatry* 12,
404–409.

Mherekumombe, M. F. (2018, April). From inpatient to clinic to home to hospice and
back: Using the "pop up" pediatric palliative model of care. *Children* (Basel) 5(5), ii.
doi:10.3390/children5050055.

Morita, T., Kuriya, M., Miyashita, M., Sato, K., Eguchi, K., & Akechi, T. (2014). Symptom burden and achievement of good death of elderly cancer patients. *Journal of
Palliative Medicine* 17(8).

Morrison, S. R. (2013). Research priorities in geriatric palliative care: An introduction
to a new series. *Journal of Palliative Medicine* 16(7).

National Guideline Alliance (UK). (2016). *End of Life Care for Infants, Children and
Young People with Life-Limiting Conditions: Planning and Management.* London:
National Institute for Health and Care Excellence.

Observatoire National de la Fin de Vie. (2013). Fin de vie des personnes agées. Sept
parcours ordinaires pour mieux comprendre les enjeux de la fin de la vie en France.
Rapport.

OECD Factbook 2009. (2009). Paris: Organisation for Economic Co-operation and
Development. Vatican City.

PAL-LIFE Expert Advisory Group. (2019). *White Book for Global Palliative Care
Advocacy.* Pontifical Academy for Life.

Pautex, S., & Vogt-Ferrier, N. (2006). Prise en charge de la douleur chronique chez la
personne âgée. *Revue Médicale Suisse* 2, 31463.

Raijmakers, N. J., van der Heide, A., Kouwenhoven, P. S., van Thiel, G. J., van Delden,
J. J., & Rietjens, J. A. (2015). Assistance in dying for older people without a serious
medical condition who have a wish to die: A national cross-sectional survey. *Journal
of Medical Ethics* 41, 145.

Robert, R., Stavinoha, P., Jones, B. L., Robinson, J., Larson, K., Hicklen, R., . . . Weaver,
M. S. (2019, April). Spiritual assessment and spiritual care offerings as a standard of
care in pediatric oncology: A recommendation informed by a systematic review of
the literature. *Pediatric Blood and Cancer* 29, e27764. doi:10.1002/pbc.27764.

Rollason, V., Bonnabry, P., & Vogt, N. (2000). Réduire la plurimédication chez la
personne âgée: du vœu pieux à des solutions applicables. *Medecine et Hygiene* 58,
818–820.

Rosenberg, A. R., Bona, K., Coker, T., Feudtner, C., Houston, K., Ibrahim, A., . . . Hays,
R. (2019, April). Pediatric palliative care in the multicultural context: Findings from
a workshop conference. *Journal of Pain and Symptom Management* 57(4), 846–855.
e2. doi:10.1016/j.jpainsymman.2019.01.005.

Rosenberg, A. R., & Wolfe, J. (2017, July). Approaching the third decade of paediatric
palliative oncology investigation: Historical progress and future directions. *Lancet
Child and Adolescent Health* 1(1), 56–67. doi:10.1016/S2352-4642(17)30014-7.

Rostad, H. M., Utne, I., Grov, E. K., Puts, M., & Halvorsrud, L. (2017, November 2).
Measurement properties, feasibility and clinical utility of the Doloplus-2 pain scale

in older adults with cognitive impairment: a systematic review. *BMC Geriatrics* 17(1), 257.

Rusalen, F., Agosto, C., Brugraro, L., & Benini, F. (2017, May). Regional paediatric palliative care model improves the quality of life of children on long-term ventilation at home. *Acta Paediatrica* 106(5), 841. doi:10.1111/apa.13769.

Scott, I. A., Hilmer, S. N., Reeve, E., Potter, K., Le Couteur, D., Rigby, D., . . . Martin, J. H. (2015, March 23). Reducing inappropriate polypharmacy: The process of deprescribing. *JAMA Internal Medicine* 175(5), 827–834.

Slater, P. J., Herbert, A. R., Baggio, S. J., Donovan, L. A., McLarty, A. M., Duffield, J. A., . . . Burr, C. A. (2018, December). Evaluating the impact of national education in pediatric palliative care: The Quality of Care Collaborative Australia. *Advances in Medical Education and Practice* 9, 927–941. doi:10.2147/AMEP.S180526.

Small, N. (2007). Living well until you die: Quality of care and quality of life in palliative and dementia care. *Annals of the New York Academy of Sciences* 1114, 194–203.

Spinewine, A., Schmader, K. E., Barber, N., Hughes, C., Lapane, K. L., Swine, C., & Hanlon, J. T. (2007, July 14). Appropriate prescribing in elderly people: How well can it be measured and optimised? *Lancet* 370.

Twamley, K., Craig, F., Kelly, P., Hollowell, D. R., Mendoza, P., & Bluebond-Langner, M. (2014, March). Underlying barriers to referral to paediatric palliative care services: Knowledge and attitudes of health care professionals in a paediatric tertiary care centre in the United Kingdom. *Journal of Child Health Care* 18(1), 19–30.

Vadeboncoeur, C., & McHardy, M. (2018, June). Benefits of early referral to pediatric palliative care for a child with a rare disease. *Pediatrics* 141(6), ii: e20173417. doi:10.1542/peds.2017-3417.

Van Lancker, A., Velghe, A., Van Hecke, A., Verbrugghe, M., Van Den Noortgate, N., Grypdonck, M., . . . Beeckman, D. (2014, January). Prevalence of symptoms in older cancer patients receiving palliative care: A systematic review and meta-analysis. *Journal of Pain and Symptoms Management* 47.

Voumard, R., Rubli Truchard, E., Benaroyo, L., Borasio, G. D., Buela, C., & Jox, R. J. (2018). Geriatric palliative care: A view of its concept, challenges and strategies. *BMC Geriatrics* 18, 220.

Weaver, M. S., Mooney-Doyle, K., Kelly, K. P., Montgomery, K., Newman, A. R., Fortney, C. A., . . . Hinds, P. S. (2019, March). The benefits and burdens of pediatric palliative care and end-of-life research: A systematic review. *Journal of Palliative Medicine*. doi:10.1089/jpm.2018.0483.

Wolfe, J., Jones, B. L., Kreicbergs, U., & Jankovic, M. (2018). *Palliative Care in Pediatric Oncology*. New York: Springer International.

World Health Organization. (2004). *Better Palliative Care for Older People*. Geneva: Author.

World Health Organization. (2011). *Palliative Care for Older People: Better Practices*. Geneva: Author.

World Health Organization. (2015). *World Report on Aging and Health*. Geneva: Author.

Zernikow, B., Szybalski, K., Hübner-Möhler, B., Wager, J., Paulussen, M., Lassay, L., . . . Schmidt, P. (2019, March). Specialized pediatric palliative care services for children dying from cancer: A repeated cohort study on the developments of symptom management and quality of care over a 10-year period. *Palliative Medicine* 33(3), 381–391. doi:10.1177/0269216318818022.

Chapter 16

International Palliative Care Advocacy

Spiritual and Secular Ethics

Katherine Pettus

Integrating palliative care delivery into primary health care is an inherently political act (in the sense that most health systems marginalize the sick and older persons by keeping their needs off the political agenda). It represents a political shift from an oligarchic monopoly of knowledge and control toward one where vulnerable individuals occupy the center of public policy. Palliative care advocacy calls on governments to deliver on their commitments to the right to palliative care as a component of the right to health, by engaging in "multi-stakeholder" efforts of workforce training and health-system strengthening, among other things. Problems could arise if, once universalized palliative care loses its distinctive holistic ethos, which is grounded in its attention to the whole person, including the family.

The now-recognized right to palliative care as a component of the right to health, which entails the right to access internationally controlled essential medicines for the relief of pain and symptoms, is a human right based on the intrinsic dignity of the person.[1] Sulmasy's claim that "Intrinsic dignity is the value that human beings have simply by virtue of the fact that they are human" (2013) echoes Dame Cicely Saunders's famous aphorism regarding hospice patients: "You matter because you are you, and you matter to the end of your life. We will do all we can not only to help you die peacefully, but also to live until you die" (Twycross, 2006). These statements echo the personalism inscribed in the Universal Declaration of Human Rights of the United Nations in 1948 and the UNESCO Declaration on Bioethics and Human Rights, which make human dignity the first principle and the inescapable grounding for all human rights (Williams, 2005; Moyn, 2011). Nations of vastly different religions, cultures, metaphysical beliefs, and historical backgrounds agreed on the secular (although universally faith based) language in these declarations. In recent years, human rights experts have confirmed a right to palliative care based on dignity, through *opinio juris*, and most recently in the Inter-American Convention on the Rights of Older Persons (Seatzu, 2015; Seatzu & Fanni, 2016; Lohman & Amon, 2015).

This genesis of this nascent body of law stipulating the right to palliative care originated in practitioner (clinical and legal) advocates who identified the *vacuum* of service provision in many parts of the world – what has been called the "abyss" in access to palliative care and pain medicines (Knaul et al., 2018). Knowing that palliative care provision can be implemented in resource-challenged as well as resource-rich countries, experts have defined member states as duty bearers and lack of provision of palliative care as violations of the rights to health and to be free of torture, cruel, and inhumane treatment. (Ezer, Lohman, & de Luca, 2018).

According to evidence gathered by the International Narcotics Control Board, the World Health Organisation, and the Lancet Commission on Palliative Care, the majority of the world's governments, as duty bearers, are anchored in this violation abyss. In 2018, the Lancet Commission reported that 25.5 million people, representing nearly half of all global deaths, died with serious health-related suffering and without palliative care. Advocates can report facts and raise ethical and political claims regarding the intrinsic dignity and human rights of persons in this abyss that are damaged by their governments' failures to ensure delivery of an affordable, essential service. The Special Rapporteur for the Convention Against Torture (Human Rights Council, 2009) has compared the suffering of persons in unrelieved severe pain – which appropriate access to palliative care could alleviate – to torture and inhumane treatment. Such entirely preventable suffering is an affront to the intrinsic dignity protected by all human rights conventions. This chapter proposes that the origin of the clinical/pharmaceutical abyss in access to palliative care is an epistemic abyss, configured by vacuums of knowledge and practice and fueled by stigma. Palliative care practitioners around the world are working to close the epistemic abyss through advocacy, workshops, trainings, and integration of palliative care modules into medical, nursing, social work, chaplaincy, and pharmacy school curricula. The multidisciplinarity of the work of repairing the epistemic abyss builds social–emotional intelligence and moves the needle of evolution toward more compassionate communities.

This shifting needle is inscribed in consensus documents drafted and approved by UN member states. These include the World Health Assembly Resolution on palliative care (67/19), which describes palliative care as "an ethical responsibility of health systems" and ethical duty of providers and refers to the "human dignity" of patients (World Health Assembly, 2014). The Inter-American Convention on the Rights of Older Persons is the first regional or global convention to explicitly define a right to palliative care and pain relief. The Astana Declaration on Primary Health Care (2018), which reaffirms the historic Alma Ata Declaration's stipulation of the universal right to access to healthcare, includes palliative care as part of the spectrum of primary healthcare. This normative framework constitutes a linguistic palliative.

The Pallium

The elements of the normative pallium discussed previously protect and promote palliative care praxis, which in turn protects the intrinsic and attributed dignity of persons experiencing severe health-related suffering. Palliative care's multidisciplinary, holistic approach places a palliative (coating of care) on the physical, psychosocial, and spiritual suffering of patients and families. In so doing, it invites beneficiaries (patients, families, and providers) to explore areas of life beyond strict utility, as defined by ordinary standards. Palliative care emphasizes the value in what is not immediately or apparently useful from an instrumental perspective (Vanistendael, 2007). In order to promote palliative care policy and ensure availability, it is necessary to demonstrate the value in what from a cost-benefit perspective is an economically "useless" service. Yet by protecting the human right to dignity at a relatively low cost, palliative care can support the resilience and sustainable development of communities and nations. By definition, sustainable development upholds dignity and builds social capital (Putnam, 2000).

In theological terms, palliative care proclaims the irreducible value of "the human being fully alive," to paraphrase Saint Irenaeus, even when extremely frail and actively dying. The dominant global health system, and most national systems, marginalize that hidden population of the dying by keeping their needs off the agenda that prioritizes reducing premature mortality. The distinct social physics of palliative care advocacy for integration of care beyond cure displaces vulnerable individuals from the margins of political attention to the center of public policy. This involves shifting the political center of gravity from a rationality of control and domination of the body and its diseases (the biomedical attempt to cure and the site of *attributed* dignity) to one of accompaniment and equality in vulnerability (palliative care and the site of intrinsic dignity). In political terms, this shift represents the evolution from an oligarchic monopoly of knowledge/power toward a radically democratic and cooperative logic that can live into the questions, to paraphrase Rilke, because they are lived in common.[2]

Palliative care is the stance of being comfortable with the unknown, a stance that leads to the development of confidence, resilience, and empowerment in patients and families receiving the best care. The fact that we are all vulnerable, all subject to suffering, old age, and death, makes strategies of avoidance through domination and control both futile and painful for all parties, particularly those outcast by serious illness. An individual's, family's, or community's capacity to embrace the unknown is transformative and evolutionary and can be expressed as the classical political virtues of magnanimity, honesty, courage, and friendship. Developed through practice and advocacy, these virtues buttress resilience and sustainable development.

The Ethics of Advocacy for Palliative Care as a Human Right

Palliative care advocacy calls on governments as duty bearers to deliver on their commitments to the right to palliative care by engaging in "multi-stakeholder" efforts of workforce training and health-system strengthening, among other things. Whether advocacy is successful in making "palliative care as available as air" – in the words of a senior Ugandan colleague – depends on the secular and spiritual ethics underlying the advocacy and implementation efforts. These ethics are radically inclusionary, as stated previously, aligning with the universal experience of pain and suffering. The danger is that as palliative care becomes "industrialized" and universally available, it will lose its distinctive holistic ethos and become just another cog in the medical industrial and global health complex. Alternatively, a clear spiritual and/or secular ethic will support practitioners to maintain and strengthen that distinctive ethos such that palliative care praxis and advocacy transform healthcare and that dominant medical industrial complex from within. Palliative care is not a "storming the gates" sort of discipline. It does not demonstrate technical wizardry of "rescue medicine" (Chapple, 2016) to save lives or reduce premature mortality; it quietly acknowledges the inherent dignity of persons with life-limiting illness, refusing to devalue brokenness, shame, or humility. In this, at its best, palliative care is radically democratic and inclusionary.

Palliative care's distinctive ethos is grounded in its attention to the whole person, including the family. Practitioners identify and attend to the "total" pain of this collective patient subjected to severe health-related suffering (Clark, 1999), which includes physical, psychosocial, and spiritual distress, many times in contexts of structural violence and injustice. The transformative power of palliative care advocacy depends upon its ability to maintain this distinctive ethos, to produce structural grace in a context of "structural sin" (Sobrino, 1997), even as it calls on governments in purely secular narratives to mainstream palliative care through primary healthcare and universal health-coverage schemes.

At the moment, palliative care is still "outsider medicine," and palliative care advocacy is countercultural and evolutionary, leaven in the dough of the global health narrative. The outsider identity derives from its emphasis – even in the public sphere – of attention to the spiritual dimension of the person, no matter what their faith or lack thereof. That said, alleviation of physical pain and distressing symptoms is the cornerstone of palliative care: relieving severe physical pain permits practitioners to approach other dimensions of distress. This requires that advocates engage with the international drug-control system, which is focused on discipline and control of substances containing "narcotic drugs," including medications, through processes of militarization and criminal justice. Proposing inclusion of "spiritual care" as "agreed language" in the

World Health Assembly resolution on palliative care precipitated a struggle, particularly with governments insisting on the modern secular value of strict separation between church and state and so deletion of the word "spiritual." The "pro-spiritual" advocates convinced them that the concept is entirely aligned with secularism, though, and prevailed. The underlying epistemological claim is that health systems that integrate secular/spiritual ethos become sites of knowledge as well as of existential accompaniment. The good news is that palliative care reconciles the physical and spiritual dimensions of persons, split in modernity at the expense of the spiritual.

Palliative care's evolutionary move is to restore balance between the two, with the dying process being a crucible for truth telling and the practice of mercy, particularly within the family. When advocates bring this extremely private and intimate process and ethos into the public square at government and multilateral meetings, they give new life to the patients and families rendered socially and civilly dead by health systems that fail to provide care beyond cure. Palliative care advocates represent those exiled voices by witnessing to the existential distress and total pain of their patients in the public square. Advocating for palliative care is subversive praxis, a stumbling block to systems fixated on treatment and cure at any cost. Once cure is no longer an option, the patients bear the physical, emotional, and spiritual costs when palliative care is not available. Advocating for them calls for *metanoia*, which in this case entails systems change.

Palliative care practitioners who advocate in the public square must take the long view, the faithful, patient (*etym*: suffering), eschatological perspective, even as the sharp thorn of untreated patient and caregiver suffering drives them relentlessly forward. Palliative care practitioners, to deploy a biblical metaphor, attend the "wedding feasts" of patients in their last months, weeks, and days, accompanying them and their families as they wrestle with diagnoses of life-limiting illness. Practitioners process with them as they go, sometimes struggling, sometimes peacefully, sometimes a chaotic mixture of both, to the final frontier, and then comfort the bereaved.

Palliative care practitioners and advocates are rarely, if ever, granted seats at the global health table. They are not honored guests in a field whose development perspective perceives palliative care advocacy as perverse. Palliative care's inability to save lives or reduce premature mortality (the bottom-line global-health goals) make it a poor candidate for philanthropic and public investment. Big funders, who could help make palliative care as available as air, inform advocates that without "measurable indicators," they cannot underwrite expanded programs. Although palliative care integrated into primary healthcare and universal coverage can slide into the "development" and measurable indicator framework, palliative care's evolutionary potential lies in its unquantifiable ethos and potential to build social capital. Palliative care advocates persist in requesting public resources to care for people who mostly don't or cannot contribute to the bottom line, as a matter of dignity and justice, not charity or aid. Such absurd petitions fly in the face of rational public policy and budgeting, particularly in this era of scarcity, security threats, and crisis. Investors and policy experts have yet to take seriously proposals that palliative care can provide social, as well as financial, returns on investment.

By contributing to knowledge building, to bridging the epistemic abyss concerning palliative care practice and the rational use of internationally controlled essential medicines, palliative care advocacy and practice nourish cosmopolitan justice. Clinicians from around the world are constantly traveling to share their skills, donating time and labor to grow the discipline, accepting lower salaries and less prestige. These efforts are often funded – at least in the case of most nongovernmental organizations (NGOs) and faith-based organizations – by generous foundation donations and individual philanthropy. Palliative care evangelism is not the traditional educational model of me filling your empty basket with my superior knowledge but of us together sharing vulnerability and wisdom in a reparative, healing attitude of humility. Together, transnational palliative care practitioners are aiming to take whole crucified continents down from the cross, to quote Fr. Jon Sobrino (1994).

Palliative care educational evangelism, which is also a form of restorative justice, is evident in many of the countries where access to internationally controlled essential medicines remains inadequate or unavailable and palliative care virtually unknown (Knaul et al., 2018). They are countries with weak health systems that are still suffering from the multigenerational historical trauma of colonialism, now perpetrated under different guises by global financial institutions and mega-corporations with incomes larger than the GDP of many of the countries. The advocacy opportunity, though, exists in the soft underbelly of the multinational institutions founded by the post–World War II visionaries and is contained in the emancipatory power of the texts, constitutions, and narratives of human rights conventions and public health. Palliative care advocacy uses those texts and narratives, including the emerging Agenda 2030 for Sustainable Development framework, to promote its unique vision of sustainable compassion.

Conclusion

The launching by the United Nations of the 2030 Agenda for Sustainable Development in 2015 – also known as the "Sustainable Development Goals" or SDGs, which have replaced the Millennium Development Goals as the global policy narrative for the next decade or so – is a piece of the palliative, the supportive context, for realization of the right to palliative care. An enormous amount of education still needs to be done to help both the voting public and policymakers understand the Sustainable Development Goals and how they can be used to promote true resilience and planetary health. Agenda 2030 is a cosmopolitan vision of person-centeredness, human rights, and environmental regeneration that can only be implemented by policymakers who have adopted an entirely different mindset than the one dominant today. In that palliative care praxis and advocacy exemplify the classical citizenship/public virtues of courage, friendship, truth telling, and magnanimity in attention to the needs of patients and families, palliative care advocacy and praxis can help transform this mindset. In fact, the paradigmatic patient, family, and multidisciplinary team are a polyphonic, democratic, mini-*polis*, to use the Greek word, where all enjoy *isegoria*, or equality of speech, which is the foundation of legitimate knowledge building.

Palliative care's alternative praxis embodies the courage to face death together, to will the good of the other – the *agape* of friendship and honest speech – or *parrhesia* (Foucault, 2005) and the generosity of giving without expecting a return. The meta-ethic of palliative care aligns with Teilhard de Chardin's definition of evolution: the process whereby the universe becomes conscious of itself. Indeed, palliative care is a discipline that demands its practitioners become conscious of themselves in order to be vulnerable to the vulnerability of the other (Caputo, 2006). By definition, becoming conscious of oneself requires the courage to deconstruct the buffered self, as philosopher Charles Taylor describes it: to be with, to live into, the truth of suffering, no matter how unpalatable or disgraceful (Taylor, 2007). Only then can clinical and social pathologies be transformed, alchemized, healed by grace, etymologically related to gratitude for Being itself. In its attention to the family, palliative care exposes and heals our interrelatedness by supporting our naturally unbuffered, or porous, selves.

The suffering others, the millions who live and die all over the world without adequate palliative care at their time of greatest vulnerability, are part of our collective selves as nations and regions in an interconnected world. Rendering entire suffering populations civilly dead by denying them palliative care violates their human rights and diminishes the resilience of the wounded body politic – the state. By approaching our shared pain with courage, friendship, skill, and honesty at the bedside *and* in the public square, practitioners and advocates honor that wounded body, taking it slowly and carefully off the cross of ignominy and indifference. Our challenge is to maintain these political/ethical/theological virtues in a spirit of faith, hope, and charity in order to prevent the assimilation of palliative care into an industrialized model of public health. Palliative care has the potential to transfigure modern healthcare systems and the larger society from mechanistic approaches that disregard the spiritual dimension to structures of grace that protect the intrinsic dignity and human rights of patients and families experiencing serious health-related suffering.

Discussion Questions

1. Discuss how palliative care is an essential component of the right to health.
2. Explain how the absence of palliative care raises issues of global health ethics.

Notes

1. Palliative care is the active holistic care of individuals across all ages with serious health-related suffering due to severe illness, especially of those near the end of life. It aims to improve the quality of life of patients, their families, and their caregivers. For the full definition, see https://hospicecare.com/what-we-do/projects/consensus-based-definition-of-palliative-care/. "Intrinsic human dignity is expressive of the inherent worth present in all humans simply by virtue of their being human. Intrinsic dignity cannot be gained or lost, expanded or diminished. It is independent of human opinions about a person's worth. It is the inherent grounding for the moral entitlements of every human to respect for one's person, one's rights, and one's equal treatment under the law in a just political order. Extrinsic or imputed dignity, on the other hand, is the assessment of the worth or status humans assign to each other or to themselves." See Pellegrino, E. D. (1988). The false promise of beneficent killing. In L. L. Emanuel (Ed.), *Regulating How We Die*, 71–91, Cambridge, MA: Harvard University Press.
2. "Be patient toward all that is unsolved in your heart and try to love the questions themselves, like locked rooms and like books that are now written in a very foreign tongue. Do not now seek the answers, which cannot be given you because you would not be able to live them. And the point is, to live everything. Live the questions now. Perhaps you will then gradually, without noticing it, live along some distant day into the answer." Letter Four (16 July 1903); Rilke, R. M., & Burnham, J. M. (1993), *Letters to a Young Poet*. Translated by M. D. Herter Norton. New York: WW Norton; originally published 1934.

References

Caputo, J. D. (2006). *The Weakness of God: A Theology of the Event*, 143. Bloomington: Indiana University Press.

Chapple, H. S. (2016). *No Place for Dying: Hospitals and the Ideology of Rescue*. New York: Routledge.

Clark, D. (1999). Total pain, disciplinary power and the body in the work of Cicely Saunders, 1958–1967. *Social Science and Medicine* 49(6), 727–736.

Ezer, T., Lohman, D., & de Luca, G. B. (2018). Palliative care and human rights: A decade of evolution in standards. *Journal of Pain and Symptom Management* 55(2), S163 – S169.

Foucault, M. (2005). *Hermeneutics of the Subject: Lectures at the Collège de France, 1981–1982*. Translated by Graham Burchell, 372. New York: Picador.

Human Rights Council. (2009, January 14). Report of the special rapporteur on torture and other cruel, inhuman or degrading treatment or punishment. Manfred Nowak, A/HRC/10/44. http://daccessdds.un.org/doc/UNDOC/GEN/G09 /103/12/PDF/G0910312.pdf?OpenElement, Accessed April 1, 2019.

Knaul, F. M., Farmer, P. E., Krakauer, E. L., De Lima, L., Bhadelia, A., Kwete, X. J., . . . & Connor, S. R. (2018). Alleviating the access abyss in palliative care and pain relief—An imperative of universal health coverage: The Lancet Commission report. *The Lancet* 391(10128), 1391–1454.

Lohman, D., & Amon, J. J. (2015). Evaluating a human rights-based advocacy approach to expanding access to pain medicines and palliative care: Global advocacy and case studies from India, Kenya, and Ukraine. *Health & Human Rights: An International Journal* 17(2).

Moyn, S. (2011). Personalism, community, and the origins of human rights. https://tif.ssrc.org/wp-content/uploads/2015/05/Personalism-Chapter.pdf, Accessed March 31, 2019.

Putnam, R. D. (2000). Bowling alone: America's declining social capital. In *Culture and Politics*, 223–234. New York: Palgrave Macmillan.

Seatzu, F. (2015). Constructing a right to palliative care: The inter-American convention on the rights of older persons. *Ius et scientia* 1(1), 25–40.

Seatzu, F, & Fanni, S. (2016). The right to palliative care: A mirage in the jurisprudence of the ECTHR and IACTHR. *Cuadernos Derecho Transnacional* 8, 5.

Sobrino, J. (1994). *The Principle of Mercy: Taking the Crucified People from the Cross*. Ossining, NY: Orbis.

Sobrino, J. (1997). The principle of mercy: Taking the crucified people from the cross. *Pro Ecclesia* 6(1), 112–114.

Sulmasy, D. P. (2013). The varieties of human dignity: A logical and conceptual analysis. *Medicine, Health Care and Philosophy* 16, 937. https://doi.org/10.1007/s11019-012-9400-1.

Taylor, C. (2007). *A Secular Age*. Cambridge, MA: Harvard University Press.

Twycross, R. (2006, March 8). A tribute to Dame Cicely Saunders, Memorial Service.

Vanistendael, S. (2007). Resilience and spirituality. *Resilience in Palliative Care: Achievement in Adversity*, 115–135.

Williams, T. D. (2005). *Who Is My Neighbor? Personalism and the Foundations of Human Rights*. Washington, DC: Cua Press.

World Health Assembly. (2014, May 24). Strengthening of palliative care as a component of comprehensive care throughout the life course. http://apps.who.int/gb/ebwha/pdf_files/wha67/a67_r19-en.pdf, Accessed April 1, 2019.

Chapter 17

Dignity Redefined
Mindfulness in Suffering

*Kathleen Benton, Ursula Bates, and
David Shannon with Michael DeLoach and
Julia DeLoach*

*As healthcare embodies the resuscitated practice of holistic medicine, heal-
ers of all disciplines search for ways to comfort progressively sick patients
with more than medicine. Virtual reality for pain, yoga, biofeedback, and
mindfulness are among some of the tactics used in this practice.*

*The focus of this chapter is the relevance of mindfulness at a patient's end
of life. Although much has been written and researched in the mindfulness
literature in relation to professional and familial caregivers with respect
to palliative care, there are just a handful of studies involving palliative
care from a patient's perspective. The authors here explore mindful suffering through the eyes of the family. Shifting tone, the authors then explain
several studies before offering some reflections born of clinical experience,
along with a clinical case vignette.*

*Mindfulness is awareness of suffering, both mental and physical. It is
presence – to acknowledge both internal and external battles. Most intimately, it is the ability to individually define reactions to external stimuli
through acknowledgment and acceptance. For someone who is ill and for
someone who is watching the demise of this ill person, mindfulness can
be healing. It is moment by moment, and it is without judgment. For the
patient and the caregiver, disease is king. Thus, control is lost. But keeping
with human nature, mindfulness gives both parties the ability to retain the
capacity to control reaction and attitude.*

Mindfulness: A Caregiver's Examination

Kathleen Benton, DrPH, MA

Daniel was handed a lot that many would not have chosen for themselves: he
was born with proteus syndrome, otherwise known as Elephant Man disease.
Others might feel forced to suffer through this wasting disease, bitter and
wanting to leave this world. Not Daniel. Daniel was diagnosed in the womb,
five months in utero, and recommended for termination. His parents were
told he would not make it a year; after he was born, he was sent home to die.

His parents were then told he would never walk, were told he would not live to age two, then age three. Despite the hurdles, Daniel soldiered on, defying doctors' predictions for 30 years. Yet, because of all of this, Daniel showed the world that the dignity of life can be a part of the most trying moments. What follows is a snapshot of one of his most difficult times and how it shaped those around him.

In a world full of immediate gratification where most of us flee from the first glimpse of pain or suffering or a shift from quality, Daniel defied social norms and clichés. He defeated death in childhood, in adolescence, and in young adulthood, choosing 100-plus surgeries, 1000-plus procedures, and thousands of hospitalizations to Band-Aid his disease and live a little longer. This man deliberately chose against passive or active euthanasia by refusing physician-assisted or individual suicide and desperately clung to life without much breath or organ function. He chose life because he loved: He loved God for giving him life, and he loved family, children, and humanity for their mere existence. Daniel defined dignity when others would have given up.

Daniel would always say that if he had to pick being born without the disease and without this family and friends, he would choose the life given to him – a remarkable statement from one who couldn't leave his bed many days because he was overcome by nausea or pain. Most of us will never experience close to a sampling of his considerable pain and anxiety in our lifetimes. Although surrounded by those who loved him, Daniel still had to face the superficial signs of social rejection, seeing it in the stares, whispers, and pointing of strangers – not to mention the truly cruel or ignorant ones who felt compelled to jeer at him, as if life were not already hard enough. Even more, he had to experience the deeper forms of social isolation, coming to terms with the fact that a relationship, a marriage with children, all he really wanted out of life, would never be available to him.

Daniel's Brother's Sentiment

Last night, cousin Katie wanted to know how you accept it. I told her: You think about Daniel's suffering being over. The last two and a half years, he has been stuck in a chair watching his one kidney fail, worrying about death and being a burden on my parents. I was only there for weeks at a time during that period, and I always thought You, Lord, would take him like a thief in the night during that time. Or maybe I did not or have never been able to consider with any seriousness You taking Daniel off of the Earth. He is such a presence, and so much life is inside of him, it is difficult to grasp the world without him. Difficult to think of that body resting for good without it being ready to jump back to life with anger and fighting.

When I write, only one title keeps coming to mind: "Must My Brother Be Forgotten," a glimpse of how I must feel that I will deal with his passing. My memory of him will fade, the accuracy will fall to some abstract points. All the details that brought it to life during the moment that was lived will be shrouded in obscurity with only a nondescript outline of the event left in its stead.

But I can reimagine the details. I just need to capture what I can write now. And I know that I must write this story. I need Your help with that. I need to be Your vessel, for You to work through me and imbue some meaning onto these days that seem so meaningless. As I sit here on a gray late January afternoon in Savannah, one of those afternoons without much definition, I muse on my brother's 29-year life, as he sits feet away struggling to breathe, with a collection of machines set up to breathe for him, filter his blood, take his heart rate, O_2 level, and blood pressure, to feed him. Machines, external organs, as Daniel would call them, allow him to press on and keep at bay that great unknown that awaits us at the end of our days.

And how can You make sense of this suffering? This is what I have thus far along those lines: What can you say when a life such as Daniel's, a life that has known such suffering, that has been so rich in that deep experience that keeps the world in its proper perspective, when a life such as his has wavered so many times before and has finally been extinguished? The futility of words feels so strong that maybe silence and unquestioning acceptance are the only proper response. But talk we must because life must go on and we must try and make some sense, draw some meaning, especially out of a life like Daniel's that seems to defy our expectations of a just world.

So, we must look at what Daniel's life has given us. This is the example of one whose suffering we cannot begin to comprehend, who in the face of this never grew bitter and continued to embrace life in a way most of us, unencumbered by chronic pain, do not take on. There are other lessons, too.

How do you mourn a loss you have been mourning since you were old enough to grasp the situation? When death never felt far away and is finally here to define the show? This can be only one more step in the mourning process.

Look at how Daniel's life has defined and has been defined by our community. I'll begin with one of the broadest factors that cannot be taken for granted. Daniel's life, whether his first 29 hours or his full 29 years, would have never have been possible in another age, and, even in this one, it is only so in a few fortunate societies.

I do not mean simply to herald modern medicine and those professionals who dedicate their time on Earth to that endeavor, the people who have cared for, operated on, counseled, and watched over Daniel during the most trying times. Modern medicine is not simply breakthroughs in science but is made up of those who are willing to pour their lives into keeping others alive.

Our society has not only given us the means to treat one with the complications of Daniel, but it has given us the will, a system set up to ensure that it is financially possible for such time and resources to be dedicated to one child's life. The imperfections of the system cannot overshadow the full picture of a system set up to care for our society's least fortunate.

So Daniel has been kept alive by our community but not only kept alive within it but welcomed, truly welcomed, into it. No opportunity has been closed to him. Rather, some have gone to great lengths, in acts that define their character, to ensure Daniel has lived as the rest of us have lived. The same opportunities to grow, to love, to befriend, to play, and to party. None of this would have been possible in many other communities, even within this same country. And I cannot overlook that and what it has meant for a life such as Daniel's.

The words come out in sparks of inspiration throughout the years, but I never took the time to record them as I should, and now they come out flowery, too positive, abstract in that they lack the concrete detail that would enable us to translate the language of my emotions to the mind of another, and unreal. Please, Lord, grant me the words I must utter when the moment comes, as tough as it may be to stare down a crowd at that time.

How should I feel these few golden alone moments I had to spend with him? I tell him I love him, and although the blanket covers his face, I can see him mouth back, "I love you, too." I ask him if he wants to talk, if he wants me to talk, or if he wants to just sit in silence. It is the latter he wishes. It would be selfish to not honor this, but what words am I leaving unsaid that will haunt me through my days?

He dials the nurse, and they come in to fill his request for Zofran and an O_2 burst. The details of keeping him alive and comfortable trump any desire I might have to try and define, bring closure to, put into words, our brotherhood.

My brother, with whom I have spent so much of this life and who, even when we are not together, still accompanies me through my days and nights. He has been given a raw deal.

Is this to be his end? Am I hiding behind language? In trying to record it, placing a camera lens between the world and me as I attempt to capture this experience rather than live it? Should I let it sink in that these are the finality of his last days on Earth? On Earth. On Earth.

We just said our goodbyes. My mom stepped out to give us our last few moments alone. I did not know quite how I would feel beforehand, not feeling tears welling up. But when I put my head on his chest, feeling his green gown brush against my cheek and hearing the vent breathe into him, hearing it through his chest, I could not hold back, especially after hearing his tears right above me. But it was that sound, the vent breathing through his chest, that will stay with me.

Now, as the darkness presses in and my mom and I prepare to leave for the day, Daniel is back under his hood again, saying he can't breathe. Having us grab a nurse in a panic and saying, in his expressive, silent way, that he needs to get some of the fluid off his peritoneal cavity.

I do not know how to handle this or how to think about it. In some ways, as odd as it may be, this feels like any of the days of old that I have spent with Daniel in the hospital room. It is hard to see these days as possibly my last with my brother, with whom I have spent every waking hour growing up, and whom I have spoken to every day on the phone, keeping track of his every move.

As we get ready to leave, Daniel has a breathing episode and we all three watch him in silent concern, arms folded across each other or holding our chins in thought. He is running a bit of a fever and does not want us to leave him on this mild February night.

Daniel had three panic attacks this morning, said he was holding the sides of the bed shaking, feeling like he could not breathe at all, ready to pass out. Worse than what we saw last night. Nothing triggered it. The panic attack woke him up. What does it feel like to wake up like that? Feeling like you can't breathe?

We said those words to each other that we needed to say. He told me, no, first asked me, if I thought he was going to die. I told him I did not know. I thought it was a strong possibility earlier, but now when I see him and his face looks so good and he has the same personality, I don't know how to think about it.

He told me he needs me to know that he is not going to die. I told him that if it is not now then, when it comes, he has to know it is okay to stop fighting.

"Do you have any idea what kind of death that would be? A terrible death. How do you just let go for that?"

I told him he "is always with me, no matter where I go. It affects how I act to those around me, how I respond to this world. My son will be Daniel, and I hope he is exactly like you."

"When you do go to get a job or have a family, make sure it is close to home. I want to be a part of their lives."

"My children will always know you."

And then, "I don't want you to go. . . . "

All of this was spoken by me and coming through from his struggled suppurations and animatedly mouthing these words that carry such weight, resounding in time.

I wish I could remember every detail. I remember minutes before it was time, thinking I would gladly sit here for 100 days, 100 years, watching over him. Love. It is not a feeling, like falling in love. It is an invisible force pressing over you, guiding your thinking and your emotions.

On the quiet, contemplative ride home with my mom, I thought, "What is this that has such a hold over us? I do not feel any changes in my body, no chemicals released, but what a strong hold it has over how I think and act."

What a strong hold love has over us.

Daniel's Suffering, From His Mother

Driving up to Augusta, the first time not in utero, I think if I had not gotten him out of his car seat because he wasn't breathing right, his heart would have stopped. That morning of torrential downpours, the second worst ever, and we zoomed up there. I carried him into the doctor's office and we took him right back and said we need to call Howell right now and get him in the ER.

That was the first time they did the colitis, slicing into each limb to try and find a vein. Imagine watching them cut on your infant. We stood outside the room, Daddy and I, and just held each other and cried. I gave you and Kathleen your snuggle bears before I left because we knew we were going to be up there a while.

After that, they put him in NICU and gave him seven units of blood because he was bleeding out of his tumor. The doctor said, "We'll get him stable and take him to a CT in the morning." That was Thursday, and we had to leave him late that night. I had cried so much I could barely open my eyes. Dr. H said, "We'll keep him through the weekend to get him more stable and then I'll operate on Monday." One doctor sat up with him all night tapping his foot to keep him up. Daniel had a lot of gas and was so weak and was so miserable.

So they operated on Monday and took off a tumor the size of a watermelon that was attached to his side. Dad came back on Wednesday, and they operated three more times. When you take off something that huge you have to do debridement because things attached start to die and you can't have that due to risk of infection. Dad would leave at a moment's notice to drive the three hours up. He would drop me off, and I would cry, and he would say he'd be right back, but sometimes it was not until the next day. They called your dad and me down to the OR because Dr. H didn't want to clip the testicle without running it by us, so we met with him outside the OR. It was scary because we did not know why the surgeon was calling to consult while Daniel was on the table.

The first pediatric orthopedist wanted to remove his feet. In Tampa, at the Shriners Hospital, we went to get a second opinion. There we were in a ward with eight children with me in a bed beside him. It was difficult to take all that young suffering. With no results after four days, a surgeon stopped me in the hall and said, "By the way, your son has a spinal cord tumor that could paralyze him."

I called my husband so upset, and he drove through the night of a terrible storm, and in the morning, he was asleep in the parking lot. We told them we would go get another opinion.

Before that time, we had to put on a steel brace to see if this would restrain the body's curvature, and they put a lift on one of his shoes because his legs had a two-inch discrepancy in length, until Dr. B operated.

The hardest operation I ever went through with Daniel was when they cauterized all the capillaries on his side to stop infections. Dr. R was giving him all the pain meds he could. Daniel was out of his mind just thanking all of the doctors. When it was over and I was headed to the car, all the sudden I had no idea where I was, just utterly disoriented. I passed this black man in the hall who said, "Smile, man." I replied, "Right now there's not too much to smile about." He returned, "You got to. It's people like you who keep us all going."

The worst time we were stuck in the hospital was when he had that terrible pain in the side when we were coming back from New Orleans. We did not even unpack the car before Daniel and I were headed to the ER, and Doctor "bag of bananas," a neurologist, put Daniel on so much medicine that he could not open his eyes. When I called her out on it, she said she was a psychopharmacologist. A psycho all right. They ended up thinking he had a tumor(?) after doing an exploratory surgery to see if there was anything in there causing that amount of pain. It could have been the ghost pain from the tumor removed when he was an infant.

When they did his second body cast at age four, that was so hard because they operated on his spinal cord tumor that Tampa had identified. I thought we were stuck because they had to put a tube deep in his chest and it kept draining and draining, which cannot be allowed to get infected because it was in his spinal canal. I thought we would never get out. We were there for two weeks. You all, of course, coming up on the weekend.

When they took us to the casting room, he had to get a cast for the bottom of his abdomen to his tilted-up chin. He was anxious as the dickens so when they cast him I brought some grape juice for him, and the only way he knew he could breathe was by swallowing grape juice. I told him if you can swallow grape juice then you can breathe. Every time they wrapped it, it grew tighter until he had sat there swallowing grape juice for two hours. We had to buy Velcro shorts to go around his body cast.

With that one, he could sit on the toilet but just needed to be assisted because he could not bend. The only problem with that one was when cousin Robert, age nine, poured sand down his body cast. I thought I was going to kill him. Dad became the official hinnie wiper, always counting the number, telling Daniel that now he owes him 197 wipes.

In the second body cast, Daniel was able to walk himself upstairs to go to bed. With the first body cast, they cut his femurs, turned his legs in, pinned them together, and took a couple inches off his left leg, his longer leg. He weighed a lot with the cast, so Dad had to lift him onto the toilet. To this day, Dad is still taking care of him, rubbing aloe vera onto his behind, red from lying in the hospital bed for days on end.

The surgery for the second body cast took 29 and a half hours, flipping him on the other side halfway through to get the entirety of the tumor and fusing his spine together.

Daniel never liked to be told he inspired someone. He would always ask what he did. There was never a choice. It was either go through all of that or die. He just did what everyone else would have done. He does not want to be a martyr, another sick child lost to disease, a fund or scholarship set up in his memory. Legacies did not interest him, only life as it is lived. Yet he must continue to teach – to teach fallen Catholics to come back to the church and resume their faith. He must teach dignity in all forms of life, even in a vessel deformed and painful, but always with joy.

The Role of Mindfulness in Patients Receiving Palliative Care

Ursula Bates, D. Clin. Psych., and David Shannon, M.Sc. Couns. Psych.

> *The experience described previously is tangible awareness of suffering. What would added mindfulness at the present moment have given to the caregivers? Research shows that caregivers suffer alongside patients, resulting in their own health problems. And as we will, most of us, become caregivers at some point, we will likewise, most of us, become the ill patient hovering near our own end of life. When nothing can be controlled but one's presence and reaction, this practice becomes even more vital.*

Current Evidence Base for Mindfulness With Patients Receiving Palliative Care

As of June 2019, there are just seven published studies that have looked at the role of mindfulness with palliative care patients. As can be seen from the studies in Table 17.1, researching the role of mindfulness in palliative care is at an early stage. However, this is beginning to grow, with four of the seven studies published since 2015. Study sample size ranged from 3 to 30. Interventions ranged from group/individual mindfulness-based stress reduction (MBSR) programs to brief practices, making it difficult to compare study outcomes. Three studies had a quantitative focus, two further studies employed a mixed-methods approach, and one was a qualitative study.

Beng et al. (2016) reported on a pilot study prior to the larger-scale Ng et al. (2016) randomized control trial, also published that year. Although the mindfulness intervention offered here was a brief five-minute breathing practice, physiological effects in terms of parasympathetic regulation were observed.

Bates's (2016) study tracked and reported on the changing narrative that patients report when developing a regular mindfulness practice. As participants became more familiar with mindfulness practice, their capacity to retain a present-moment focus orientation increased and they appeared to ruminate less. They reported greater ability to self-regulate in the face of their symptom burden and an increased capacity to retain a sense of identity. This goes to the heart of what has been termed "secondary suffering" (Burch & Penman, 2013): our reactions to unpleasant experiences that compound them and make them even more challenging.

Bergmark Kudan and Edlund (2016) adopted a mixed-methods case-study approach to explore the effects of a seven-day mindfulness training program in relation to symptom burden. As symptom burden remains a central focus of

Table 17.1 Author, Study Design, Participant Number.

Author (Year)	Study Design	Partici-pants (n =)	Intervention	Region
Beng et al. (2016)	Quasi-experiment	3	5-minute mindful breathing practice	Malaysia
Ng, Lai, Tan, Sulaiman, and Zainal (2016)	Quasi-experiment	30	5-minute mindful breathing practice	Malaysia
Bates (2016)	Mixed methods	6	Individual MBSR-based 8-week program	Ireland
Bergmark Kudan and Edlund (2016)	Mixed methods	6	7-day program	Sweden
Van den Hurk, Schellekens, Molema, Speckens, and van der Drift (2015)	Mixed methods	16	MBSR 8-week group program	Holland
Tsang, Mok, Lam, and Lee (2012)	Quasi-experiment	28	Body scan meditation	China (Hong Kong)
Chadwick, Newell, and Skinner (2008)	Qualitative (interpretative phenome-nological analysis)	5	6-week program	United Kingdom

palliative care, recording outcomes in relation to scores of commonly experienced symptoms is well warranted. They found a beneficial effect of mindfulness practice in relation to patients' subjective experience of symptom burden. Using the Edmonton Symptom Assessment Scale (ESAS; Bruera et al., 1991), patients with just seven days of mindfulness training reported lower scores on the ESAS. The ability to relax and become calm was also reported as a significant outcome.

Van den Hurk et al. (2015) specifically chose to focus on the effects of mindfulness training in relation to patients with advanced lung cancer. They note that participation in MBSR instigated positive change in patients. Tsang et al. (2012) researched the effects of playing a 45-minute "body scan meditation" on patients receiving palliative care after an individualized one-to-one session lasting 90 minutes. Patients were followed up after one week and again after one month. Gains in terms of pain reduction and vitality were greatest after one month.

Finally, Chadwick et al. (2008) pioneered research in this area and offered insights into patients' experiences of mindfulness using the methodology of interpretative phenomenological analysis (IPA; Smith et al., 2009). Chadwick et al. (2008) reported on patient improvement in body awareness and mood. Participants also found the group process and hospice environment supportive, suggesting that context for mindfulness training may also play a role.

Although these studies are tentative due to limitations in numbers and methodology, they are reporting a trend toward stress reduction, reduction in perceived symptom burden, and greater self-regulation. Overall, no increased distress was reported, and the method with adaptations was acceptable to palliative patients. Latorraca, Martimbianco, Pachito, Pacheco, and Riera (2017) conducted a systematic review of mindfulness in palliative care and reported that only two studies showed significant differences: one in terms of stress management and one for quality of life. Overall, they noted that all the studies were at risk for bias.

Considerations When Introducing Mindfulness to Patients in Palliative Care

In Our Lady's Hospice and Care Services, the authors have delivered MBSR in group day hospice since 2005. In 2012, we extended the service to include individual mindfulness sessions with patients. In addition, since 2012, we have trained some 65 staff members in MBSR. To support staff and patients, we hold two open 30-minute sitting practice sessions per week. Our experiences of introducing patients to mindfulness within a large urban (Dublin, Ireland) palliative care center have revealed several organizational as well as patient-specific considerations.

- A person's capacity to "attend" is a prerequisite to developing greater mindfulness. Although mindfulness is a natural capacity, the deliberate/ intentional focusing of attention is a cognitively demanding task. Therefore, cognitive impairment, particularly in terms of the "alerting" and "orienting" of attention, may be a limiting factor for some patients.
- Although the breath is often used as a focus of attention early on in mindfulness training, patients who have breathing difficulties should be closely monitored and offered alternative choices (e.g., "feet-on-floor" or other neutral focus) about where to focus their attention.
- The arc of MBSR and mindfulness-based cognitive therapy (MBCT) programs offers a helpful template in adapting mindfulness on an individual or group basis where time may not allow for the standard 2.5-hour sessions each week for eight weeks. The first four weeks of MBSR/MBCT focus on stabilizing attention while noticing habits such as "mind wandering" and operating in "automatic pilot" mode. The

second half of the eight-week program then more specifically encourages opening to and "turning toward" difficulty. We have found placing the emphasis on stabilizing attention by returning to the body and breath to be a helpful focus in initial individual and day hospice group sessions, given the inherent instability and uncertainty surrounding serious illness.

- Existing levels of anxiety/depression should be monitored; as mindfulness leads to greater awareness of all aspects of experience, this may lead to a subjective increase in anxiety. Although this is normal, this is one of the reasons those offering mindfulness training need to embody the "attitudinal foundations" (Kabat-Zinn, 2013) of mindfulness practice that participants are being encouraged to bring to their experience. This is the "heartfulness" aspect of mindfulness, without which the practice may well be experienced as stress inducing rather than one of stress reduction.

In 2016, eight palliative care patients participated in a qualitative study (Bates, 2016) on mindfulness in palliative care. The following is an extract from an interview with a palliative care patient who had attended individual and group mindfulness sessions in day hospice over 12 weeks.

Jason, aged 55, had a diagnosis of prostate cancer, which was now advanced. He was struggling with symptoms of tinnitus, pain, and fatigue. He was an engineer by profession, married with two teenage children. He was referred to psychology, as he was very quiet in day hospice, and the staff were concerned that he was depressed. He was not interested in therapy but agreed to engage in mindfulness. The discipline and focus of mindfulness appealed to his scientific mind.

Jason's normal coping strategies, working hard and providing for his family, had failed in the face of his illness. "I crawl under the duvet . . . in the foetal position and I would wait hopefully for it to pass, but there is not much left for you then." At one point he had seriously thought of suicide. "Yeah sometimes you can actually be very morbid and often wish it was over, you know, playing the waiting game."

As he developed a practice using the body scan, he gained a broader field of awareness. His focus on his tinnitus lessened and his ability to manage his hospitalizations increased. He was in the same hospital room with the same procedures but experienced it differently.

"I felt I had no control over myself when I was institutionalised, because it is like going to prison, with the mindfulness you gain a sense of control. You are not on your own, and you are not so much in charge of anything like that, but you have an identity rather than being another patient or part of the furniture let's say. You keep your identity."

Gradually, by session, five his mood lifted. Jason found that using the key words of the loving-kindness meditation enabled him to cope with depression. "So when I feel that coming on, when I feel the emotional wave, I say the three words (may I be happy, may I be safe, and may I be well) and it's like a light switch, it just brings a smile to my face."

By session eight, his narrative cognitive self-processing had reduced, and he talked less about the past, less about external events or the future. "I have stopped forecasting things then you say that's too much for me. But when you are in the moment you can sort of react more to it, and say 'I'm up for it, I don't have to plan for it, I can do it.'"

Discussion Questions

1. What are some mindfulness practices used in PC?
2. How can mindfulness practices as a routine in palliative care impact patients' end-of-life care?

References

Bates, U. (2016). Mindfulness in palliative care. Doctorate in Clinical Psychology thesis, National University of Ireland, Galway, Ireland.

Beng, T. S., Ahmad, F., Loong, L. C., Chin, L. E., Zainal, N. Z., Guan, N. C., . . . Meng, C. B. C. (2016). Distress reduction for palliative care patients and families with 5-minute mindful breathing: A pilot study. *American Journal of Hospice and Palliative Medicine* 33(6), 555–560.

Bergmark Kudan, M., & Edlund, P. (2016). Experience of a mindfulness program and its impact on symptoms in patients with cancer in a palliative phase. Advanced Masters dissertation, Sophia Hemmet University, Sweden.

Bruera, E., Kuehn, N., Miller, M. J., Selmser, P., & Macmillan, K. (1991). The Edmonton Symptom Assessment System (ESAS): A simple method for the assessment of palliative care patients. *Journal of Palliative Care* 7(2), 6–9.

Burch, V., & Penman, D. (2013). *Mindfulness for Health: A Practical Guide to Relieving Pain, Reducing Stress and Restoring Wellbeing*. Hachette UK.

Chadwick, P., Newell, T., & Skinner, C. (2008). Mindfulness groups in palliative care: A pilot qualitative study. *Spirituality and Health International* 9(3), 135–144.

Kabat-Zinn, J. (2013). *Full Catastrophe Living: How to Cope with Stress, Pain and Illness Using Mindfulness Meditation*. London: Piatkus.

Latorraca, C. D. O. C., Martimbianco, A. L. C., Pachito, D. V., Pacheco, R. L., & Riera, R. (2017). Mindfulness for palliative care patients: Systematic review. *International Journal of Clinical Practice* 71(12).

Ng, C. G., Lai, K. T., Tan, S. B., Sulaiman, A. H., & Zainal, N. Z. (2016). The effect of 5 minutes of mindful breathing to the perception of distress and physiological responses in palliative care cancer patients: A randomized controlled study. *Journal of Palliative Medicine* 19(9), 917–924.

Smith, J. A., Flowers, P., & Larkin, M. (2009). *Interpretative Phenomenological Analysis: Theory, Method and Research*. Thousand Oaks, CA: Sage.

Tsang, S. C. H., Mok, E. S. B., Lam, S. C., & Lee, J. K. L. (2012). The benefit of mindfulness-based stress reduction to patients with terminal cancer. *Journal of Clinical Nursing* 21(17–18), 2690–2696.

Van den Hurk, D. G., Schellekens, M. P., Molema, J., Speckens, A. E., & van der Drift, M. A. (2015). Mindfulness-based stress reduction for lung cancer patients and their partners: Results of a mixed methods pilot study. *Palliative Medicine* 29(7), 652–660.

Conclusions

Renzo Pegoraro

In recent years, a growing interest in palliative care has emerged for the purposes of better responding to the needs of patients – that is, the physical, psychological, and spiritual needs of the seriously ill and those who are in the final stages of their lives.

The path outlined in the chapters in this book offers an important perspective to promote palliative care and encourage medical congruence.

Unfortunately, in the last decades, medicine has become more and more specialized, sectoral, and focused on a part of the person's body, losing sight of a comprehensive and unitary vision of the sick person as a whole. Medicine as it is currently practiced has developed increasingly sophisticated diagnostic and therapeutic technologies, focused on the detection of specific parameters and markers and offering targeted therapies but neglecting what cannot be measured and treated: the soul of the person, his or her inner life, the fears and hopes of the patient, his or her relationship with family members and other significant people.

What therefore emerges is the need to recover and cultivate a holistic, person-centered perspective and promote attention to a human sense of the experience of vulnerability and mortality and of care at the time of illness and death.

In this social and welfare effort that involves everyone, from patients, families, and healthcare professionals to health institutions, citizens, social networks, and the mass media, religions can play an important role in understanding the existential meaning of the experience of suffering and death, their expression in social rituals, openness to transcendence, and concrete forms of care and accompaniment.

Religions have always been deeply involved in the reality of death and, even more so today, they are challenged by new situations, old problems that have partly changed or others that are completely new. Reflection and practice in religious traditions can – and perhaps must – help us to understand the meaning of the end of our lives and of our mortality; they can and must help us to take a more focused approach to the reality of pain, suffering, and fear of advancing disease and approaching death; they can and must help us to understand a hope that goes beyond this life, to try to accompany the end of this life in the most humane and dignified way possible.

A sincere dialogue and effective collaboration among all those involved and reference to the cultural and religious traditions present can help us develop palliative care for all, palliative care early and simultaneously for every serious disease and in the dying process.

All stakeholders are involved in this effort with important and useful recommendations as proposed in the *White Book for Global Palliative Care Advocacy* by the Pal-Life expert advisory group of the Pontifical Academy for Life.

> The new opportunities to expand palliative care globally offer the chance for "palliative care for all." Addressing the challenges and creating a clear vision requires engagement of all the stakeholders with "new responsibilities" which are individual and collective. As healthcare professionals, we need to be trained in palliative care and develop competency in accompanying the dying. As citizens, collectively, we need to advocate for palliative care integration into our medical care systems locally and nationally creating models of humane, compassionate, competent care for those who are dying.
>
> (Foley, 2018, 154)

Reference

Foley, K. (2018). Accompanying life in the passage of death. In V. Paglia & R. Pegoraro (Eds.), *Accompanying Life: New Responsibilities in the Technological Era*. Rome: PAV.

Index

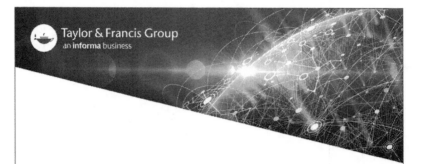